I0415433

Healthy Eating Mindset

Complete Step-by-Step Guide on How to Obtain the
Best Mindset for Healthy Eating to Create a Healthy
Relationship with Food and Feel Great Physically and
Mentally

Improve Yourself Series Book 1

GARRETT REDFIELD

TABLE OF CONTENTS

INTRODUCTION

With all the fad diets and intense exercise regimens in the world today, developing a new, healthy relationship with food may seem overwhelming—but the aim of this book is to simplify that process in a way that prioritizes your mindset rather than promote an ideal body weight or strict diet plan. This instructional book will guide you to a new healthy eating mindset through easy, personalized steps so that you can feel good mentally and physically about what you eat. A healthy mindset is an all-important foundation for the relationship that connects food, body, and spirit—and the goal of this book is to help you build this foundation so that you can face whatever goal you have with confidence and determination.

The following chapters will discuss the planning and preparation phases to help you develop your new healthy mindset, explain the connection between eating healthy and feeling good, and provide you with several methods to develop and maintain your new healthy eating mindset. In this way, all the information provided in this book will equip you to reshape your habits and the way you think about eating before you embark on any challenging diets or exercise programs. Provided with this information in advance, you will be able to enjoy a stable and quick transition into whatever lifestyle changes you would like to achieve. In addition, the advice included within this book should prove useful in case you need to refer back to it in the future, as progress toward a new mindset is a journey and not an instant exchange.

There are plenty of books on this subject on the market—thanks a lot for choosing this one! Every effort was made to ensure that it is full of as much useful information as possible. Please enjoy! In addition, if you find this book helpful or enjoyable, consider leaving a review on Amazon to let other readers know!

CHAPTER 1: SET YOURSELF UP FOR SUCCESS

One of the most difficult hurdles to overcome when taking on any lifestyle change is the question of where to start, especially when that change is centered on developing a new mindset. That is why the crucial first step of developing a new healthy eating mindset concerns establishing a structured, concrete foundation upon which you can build all later ideas about your relationship with food. It is important not to overlook the influence that these initial moments can have on your entire healthy mindset journey—you might, in fact, even say that it sets the tone for all later developments.

The most important aspects of the planning and preparation stage involve setting yourself up for success. These steps will ensure that you have a strong baseline to fall back upon in case you find any difficulties in transitioning into your new mindset. After all, setbacks and slip-ups are part of what it is to be human! This foundation will help you get back on track easily without feeling that you have lost any progress. The time taken to set yourself up for success will help make every step on your mindfulness journey seem more realistic—in a sense creating a map of where you want to go and how you plan to get there.

Identify Your Resources

Before embarking upon your journey toward a new healthy eating mindset, be sure that you are aware of all the resources available to you. Depending upon your location and region, you may have a plethora of healthy eating options—including organic markets, vegan restaurants, or culinarily-gifted friends willing to take this journey with you. If you are unsure what kind of resource you have in your area, take a moment to do a bit of research and ask yourself the following questions:

• Am I willing to expand my options geographically to meet the needs of my new healthy eating mindset?

• Can I be flexible with the resources I want to include in my healthy eating mindset journey?

• How can I be open to new experiences and new resources in my area, such as farmer's markets or unfamiliar restaurants?

• Even at a regular supermarket or grocery store, can I orient my grocery shopping around a healthy eating mindset, such as purchasing more fresh produce and organic ingredients?

Be sure to make the most of the resources immediately available to you while also continually looking for new resource opportunities in order to maximize the potential of your area. For example, if you live in a rural area with few organic, vegetarian, or vegan restaurant regions in your neighborhood, take advantage of local produce at farmer's markets and see if there is a nearby town where you can meet needs otherwise unsatisfied by local producers. On the other hand, if you live in a suburban area and are unaware of any local farmer's markets, make use of organic supermarkets in your area and experiment with nearby restaurants' organic and vegetarian menu options. You can even make Saturday mornings special by dedicating them to taking trips to markets that would usually be out of the way in your regular commute.

Whatever resources you find in your area and however you decide to use them, try to plan your week around these resources. In this way, you can create a structured schedule to help guide you through your coming journey. Consider doing your regular grocery shopping on the same day every week, and experiment with weekend outings to either farmer's markets or special restaurants, as mentioned above. In the beginning, you may find it easiest to just add these new resources to your current grocery and restaurant options—but as you advance in your healthy eating mindset, it may serve you best to transition to these new resources alone completely.

Resources can also include more than just sources of food and ingredients. For instance, this book acts as a resource for information on healthy eating mindsets. You can also seek out informative resources to supplement this book, such as reading new and exciting lifestyle articles about healthy eating mindsets, new recipes, or ways to alter and improve your diet. Additionally, there may be lifestyle groups in your area where like-minded individuals can get together to discuss their mindfulness goals or try new eateries to expand their resources. Creating a social aspect of your healthy eating mindset can allow you to develop new habits and learn new mindfulness techniques. You can even branch out past mindful eating interests into other activities, such as meditation and yoga groups or cooking classes. Not only will social resources provide you with motivation and new information, but they will also play the all-important role of making your lifestyle changes fun! Although a lot of mindfulness centers on you as an individual and your internal thoughts or actions, connecting with others over mindfulness techniques and new relationships with food will nourish the private developments in your life. This creates a positive feedback loop, where you are bolstered emotionally and encouraged to continue each time that you interact with like-minded individuals. These positive reinforcements will help strengthen your desire to develop your healthy eating mindset, which will preemptively establish support and encouragement for when you find yourself less motivated to stick to your new habits, such as your diet plan.

Create a Flexible Diet Plan

A major distinguishing trait between a traditional diet plan and the healthy eating mindset that you are aiming for is the flexibility available. Whereas regular diets severely limit what you are allowed to eat and often prioritize a one-size-fits-all eating regimen, a healthy eating mindset has no strict nutritional limits and only requires you to eat what makes you feel healthy and satisfied with your relationship with food. As you develop your own unique healthy eating mindset, you will no doubt find ways to personalize your diet to best suit your individual needs. At the beginning of your journey though, you may find it helpful to start from a basic diet plan that you can adjust according to the resources you have available in order to create a sense of structure in your healthy eating transition. This book's suggested diet plans can be followed by anyone regardless of geographical location or economic means, and they act as simple guidelines rather than strict limitations. We will go further into these non-restrictive diet plans and how to personalize them in Chapter 3: Creating Your Healthy Mindset.

The organic option: Thanks to the establishment of organic grocery chains and USDA-regulated labeling, maintaining an organic-oriented diet has never been easier! Switching to an all-organic diet can be a rather simple step—since almost all food products are available in organic options. Additionally, you can supplement store-bought organic groceries with local produce and animal products. It is easy to ask farmers about their crop-raising techniques, on the local level, to ensure that their produce was not treated with pesticides or other harsh chemicals. The clean and healthful qualities of organic food can provide you with a wholesome and rewarding feeling both in your mind and body.

The vegetarian/vegan option: Although you can develop a perfectly healthy diet that incorporates meat and animal products such as dairy, some readers may wish to limit their diets to fruits, vegetables, and grains. The benefit of vegetarian and vegan diets is that they provide an extra layer of mindfulness to your healthy eating mindset—that is, it can help you to meditate on other aspects of food production outside of your immediate sphere of influence. Many vegetarians and vegans maintain their diet due to concerns of animal cruelty or pollution as a by-product of meat production. This may be helpful for you when developing your own healthy eating mindset, but you should be sure to work your way up to any new diet slowly, as any major lifestyle change can prove difficult. If you were a regular meat eater prior to adopting a healthy eating mindset as a goal, try to exclude one type of animal product at a time while experimenting with other ingredients and recipes. This way, you can make a comfortable transition to your new diet. Otherwise, you may find yourself unsure of how to prepare tofu or end up eating the same salad every day!

The garden-to-table option: This diet option may require more research or effort than the previous two, but it can also be infinitely more rewarding and edifying from a healthy eating mindset standpoint. The garden-to-table approach consists of the same organic and produce-oriented staples as the other options, but it is differentiated by its emphasis on local or self-grown foods. The "garden" may be your own, a friend's, a community garden, or the garden of a local farmer. In any case, this option helps increase your mindfulness of the production and consumption cycle of food and highlights your role in the food cycle of your local community. Choosing to grow your own food can also help you create a brand new positive connection with your diet; since you are putting hard work and effort into growing your own fruits and veggies, you will feel especially rewarded and successful when you get to harvest and eat the delicious food! You can also incorporate the garden-to-table method into either of the two other diet options, and you can help create mindfulness by doing something as simple as growing herbs in a small indoor pot—you don't need to have a huge backyard and expansive vegetable garden to learn about the virtues of growing your own food!

Whichever diet plan you choose to start with, and whether you strive to stick closely to the basic plans outlined here or choose to hybridize the ideas into our own special diet plan, it is important to understand that the diet is only a very small part of your mindful eating growth. Of course, having a diet to fall back on can make it much easier for you, but the true value of a diet is its ability to make you rethink your relationship to food. Rather than thinking of food as a necessity to survive, as something that you eat without much thought, or as something to act as a means to an end—like the perfect body—instead think of it as a special part of your life that brings value to you, both physically and spiritually. What that value is exactly is up to you. Hopefully, your new diet plan helps you evaluate for yourself what kinds of value you wish to receive from your meals and how to maximize and appreciate that value.

As a warning, do not place too much value on your diet plan of choice. Although diets can be a wonderful and effective tool in reshaping your relationship with food, they can also cause you to develop unhealthy eating habits when used in the wrong way. Consider a strict and highly limited diet that requires you to cut out most of your old food choices in favor of a single type of food product. There are several ways that this diet could negatively impact your physical and emotional health. First, you may become frustrated with the extreme restrictiveness of the diet and come out of it with a negative experience that colors your future interactions with health plans, perhaps biasing you against such lifestyle changes. Another negative outcome is the possible degradation of your physical health due to a lack of necessary vitamins or minerals. This would not only directly impact your body, but it would also hurt you emotionally and spiritually, as the mind is interconnected with the body. Finally, you could develop an unhealthy view of your body and food, placing the aesthetic outcome of a diet above the holistic and internal good that could be cultivated through healthy eating. Such an unhealthy view would severely damage your body image until you reached an "ideal" body shape, while possibly leaving permanent emotional issues concerning your relationship with food and your physical appearance. It could also lead to nutrient depletion, as mentioned in the second outcome example. Although these negative outcomes are not inevitable when undertaking a restrictive diet, they are extremely common dangers. That is why mindful eating purposefully keeps its distance from fad diet plans and extreme weight loss methods such as fasting.

Instead of punishing your body or thinking of diets as cure-alls for body image issues, healthy eating mindsets ask you to reconsider your view of the purpose of diets. The diet plans mentioned above are not meant to be short-term methods of losing weight or detoxifying the body but rather as long-term lifestyle changes that can help improve your relationship with food and your view of your physical and mental health. This is why mindful eating emphasizes feeling good rather than looking good, as the latter goal often prioritizes skin-deep improvement at the cost of your emotional and spiritual health. Healthy eating mindsets and healthy habits start working from the inside out, tending to your internal needs and, in turn, helping you to feel good on the outside as well.

Friends and Family: A Network of Support

In addition to resources and diet plans, an incredibly stabilizing force in your development of a healthy eating mindset is the network of support available to you. By simply telling your friends and family about the journey you are undertaking, you can create accountability for yourself as you go forward. As humans are social creatures, we crave the support and approval of those close to us. We also benefit tremendously from positive feedback and simple reminders.

Consider the following example: Imagine a woman named Claire wants to improve her eating mindset, and so she chooses to change her diet and begins using mindfulness techniques to improve her relationship to food. However, she does not feel that she sees the desired results as soon as she thought she would. Since she never told anyone that she wanted to create a healthy eating mindset, she quietly gives up and returns to her former eating habits. Meanwhile, another woman on the same mindfulness journey, Miranda, told several friends about her goal when she first started. When, a few days into her new diet and mindfulness practice, she began to feel less motivated about her goal, she considered giving up. However, she met with a friend over coffee, and her friend asked her about her healthy eating mindset growth. Miranda admitted that she was not feeling very confident about it, but her friend encouraged her, saying, "It sounds like such a good idea! I might even join you!" With support from her friend, Miranda continues to develop her healthy eating habits and mindfulness.

Even if you find that your close friends and family do not have much interest in healthy eating mindsets, thanks to modern technology you can turn to online groups and social media to enrich your mindful social circle. In fact, you may even find it easier to share your mindfulness journey with people online, since you are more likely to find other mindful eaters through specific websites and forums. In addition to this, there are plenty of blogs and videos dedicated to mindfulness, healthy eating, self-improvement, and flexible diet plans available online. On top of the friendship and support that you can garner from online resources, you can also take your journey public through your own social media so that you can actively track your development and share your discoveries with others! You can never tell when you may aid someone in a mindfulness journey of their own or when an enthusiastic comment on your social media update will inspire you to take your healthy eating journey to the next level!

Being open and vulnerable with others will show them that you take your mindful eating journey very seriously and would deeply appreciate their support. More importantly, it will help you understand and accept your place in the larger community in which you exist. Of course, your focus is on improving your relationship with food, but this relationship touches and affects every aspect of your life. It has been said that eating is an inherently social activity—friends get together at restaurants and families have meals together—and the symbol of "breaking bread" is one of the most deeply meaningful actions among groups of people. By informing others about your intentions and asking for support, you acknowledge the inherently social aspect of a personal journey based around food. As we mentioned earlier, your food choices place you within a larger sphere of food production and consumption, and this journey likewise asks you to reevaluate food's place within your social circle. By beginning with mindfulness centered on what you consume, you are prepared to "think outwards" and apply that mindfulness to social activities related to food and, later on, all aspects of your life. In this way, the decision to be open and ask for support from friends and family strengthens the social connections you already have while preparing you to build new ones as your mindfulness journey commences.

As you can see, even one positive voice of support

can be the deciding factor to continue when you feel like giving up. By telling all of your friends and family, you create a safety net for when you feel doubt or disappointment. Like Miranda's friend, they might even join you on your mindfulness journey! Furthermore, if you let your friends know what exactly your goals are and how you plan to achieve them, they can help you on your way! They may know a restaurant that offers healthy options to align with your new diet, or they may volunteer to go to farmer's markets with you to do your grocery shopping. All types of journeys benefit from fellow travelers, and the journey to a healthy eating mindset is no different.

The Many Paths to a Healthy Eating Mindset

There has been a landslide of information introduced to you in this first chapter. However, you should not feel overwhelmed by any means! One of the tenets of mindfulness is the reminder to take comfort in what you are capable of in the present rather than worrying about everything you think you must do. In that light, remind yourself that not everything included in this book will fit into your lifestyle—the goal of this introductory chapter, in particular, is to present you with many potential techniques and methods that you can use on your journey toward establishing a mindful relationship with food. In a sense, there are many pathways that you can take toward a healthy eating mindset, and even within those several paths, you have the ability to choose which of the manifold steps you want to take and in which direction.

You should also keep in mind that there is no single definition of a healthy eating mindset. Everyone has their own deeply personal relationship with food, and the goal of developing a healthy eating mindset of your own depends entirely upon what you want to get out of your journey. There is no perfect solution to unhealthy eating—we should only mindfully aim for improvement in some way. Each person who reads this book will take away a different conclusion and subsequently embark on a unique journey that leads to a perfectly individual end. Part of the mindful emphasis in a healthy eating mindset is remembering to focus on your individual needs and growth rather than comparing yourself to others. This realization that your character will result in a lifestyle that cannot be compared to anyone else's is at the very heart of mindfulness. In turn, this realization will help you create a sense of detachment from worry, envy, or shame. The journey toward a healthy and mindful relationship with food never really ends, so it is important to develop a sense of calm and to feel at peace with wherever you are at in your own journey and where you might end up.

That being said, as you prepare to embark on your journey, be sure to ask yourself what goals you wish to set for your new healthy eating mindset. Having several small goals will make your improvement feel more tangible, and each time you meet a goal, you will feel accomplished and proud of your journey so far. There are many different outcomes possible within the umbrella term of a "healthy eating mindset," so you should work out ahead of time exactly what you wish to accomplish on your journey. A simple place to start is to ask yourself what aspect of a healthy eating mindset you wish to place the most emphasis upon: the physical or mental? If you wish to focus on the physical outcomes of a healthy eating mindset, you may set goals such as the following:

• I will put healthy food into my body so that I can be physically healthier, have more energy, and live longer.

• I will improve my relationship with food so that I can alter my diet and be more nutritious, thereby losing weight in a healthy, mindful way.

Notice the way these verbal goals are structured: There are both confidence and decisiveness in the way they are stated, and they outline the actions you will take as well as the outcomes that you expect. These goals can be personalized and narrowed further to suit your needs in order to give you direction on your mindfulness journey. Likewise, you can develop goals that focus on the mental health benefits of a healthy eating mindset:

• I will redefine my relationship with food so that I can feel better emotionally about what I consume.

• I will meditate on what I eat so that I can gain a better understanding of my role in the cycle of production and consumption.

• I will learn to appreciate the relationship between food and the body so that I can improve my body image and learn to love myself in whatever shape I am.

Goals like these will help guide you throughout your journey and provide you with a map, in a sense, of ways to develop your healthy eating mindset. You may or may not wish to share your goals with others because they can be deeply personal, but if you do choose to share them, remember that this is a way to be open and vulnerable with your friends and family, who in turn can support you as you work toward achieving these goals. With goals that focus on mental improvement, in particular, talking through the doubts or worries you may have can help provide clarity on your position as you develop your healthy eating mindset. In this way, you begin your journey already acknowledging and working with the connection between mind and body—this will aid in your understanding as you reevaluate your relationship to food not only in a physical way but also as a relationship that affects your mental health.

Now that you have considered your foundations in resources, diet options, support networks, and unique pathways and goals, you are ready to begin your journey toward a healthy eating mindset. This preparation has set you up for success so that you can acknowledge where you are beginning from, decide where you want to end up, as well as consider the ways that you can get to your end goal. Most importantly though, it should familiarize you with the purpose of a healthy eating mindset versus traditional diet plans and equip you with the understanding that a healthy mindset is own of growth, self-forgiveness, and perpetual improvement that focuses on your health both on the inside and outside. Now that you are prepared for success, it is time to dive into the act of incorporating mindfulness into your life so that you can improve your relationship with food in a way that benefits your mental and physical health.

CHAPTER 2: UNDERSTANDING THE MIND AND BODY

To those unfamiliar with mindfulness techniques and productive meditation, a mere mindset change may seem irrelevant when considering lofty goals of physical self-improvement. However, mindfulness has been practiced for centuries as a companion to physical improvement due to the powerful connection between the mind and body. Mindfulness is perhaps most well-recognized as part of the practice of yoga. Few people will deny the physical benefits of regular yoga practice, and the mental benefits are also widely appreciated. These mental effects stem from the mindfulness practices of relaxation, deep breathing, focus, and connection that are emphasized in yogic practice. Many yogis practice in large classes in order to acknowledge their connection with others, and students often benefit from the calm guidance of a teacher. Together, all these factors work to bring mindfulness to your actions—it is an incredibly rewarding experience, which is why yoga is so popular in Western countries today, even though it developed long ago in the continent of Asia.

Many people across the world practice mindfulness today. Although the individual has his or her own reason for pursuing a more mindful lifestyle, the meditations of mindfulness work to bring disparate ideas and actions together—this connection with others and with the world is important to mindfulness. As you acknowledge your own strengths and weaknesses, your own goals and setbacks, you gain a better understanding of the universe at large, which nourishes your soul in turn. This growing sense of connection and inner peace has led mindfulness to become a popular practice in regular people's daily routines, an important tool in the arsenal of holistic physical trainers, and also a method of mental growth and self-improvement as used by many psychologists today—but it has not always been this way. In order to understand the undeniable benefits of mindfulness and learn why it should be at the heart of any self-improvement journey, we should consider its history and original purposes.

A Brief History of Mindfulness

The practice we know today as mindfulness has its roots in eastern religion as a spiritual practice. Hinduism is widely considered to be the oldest religion in the world that is still practiced today, and it has had an immeasurable influence on the world's population, including people who practice other religions. It is a religion with no single founder—in fact, Hinduism did not even exist as a single coherent religion until the British began referring to various Vedic traditions in India and surrounding regions as "Hinduism"—and many distinct schools of thought. However, mindfulness has been an important part of Hinduism for thousands of years, and some experts even argue that the history of Hinduism is itself a history of mindfulness. This is true in part, although Buddhism has also had major impacts on the practice. One thing to take note of is the fact that Buddhism itself is one of the aforementioned religions that has been influenced by Hinduism, but it still must be considered an entirely separate and unique tradition. In this way, Buddhism has uniquely affected mindfulness— referred to as Sati in the Buddhist tradition—as it branched away from Hindu beliefs and practices. A key difference between Hinduism and Buddhism is the importance of Vedic texts; while Hinduists base their practices around reading these ancient religious texts, Buddhist reject the need to study the texts and instead focus on internal wisdom. Most yoga studios and meditation leaders in America today subscribe to mindfulness that has developed in the Buddhist tradition, particularly Zen Buddhism, although at the end of a yoga session you are also likely to hear the familiar Hindu greeting, "Namaste." The reason for this mixed influence is due to the religions' overlapping histories and shared beliefs. In particular, both Hinduism and Buddhism are concerned with the concept of dharma, which is an idea that is difficult to translate but often given the meaning of "living in harmony with the universe." This concept of dharmic living is vital to mindful practices, and it has been interpreted in many ways over the years. Some people translate dharma into their lives as "being at peace with the world" or "loving who you are as you love others." Depending on your own personal philosophies, you will take a unique meaning from the concept of dharma in order to guide your mindfulness practice.

The dharmic emphasis in Buddhism is concerned with attaining enlightenment, or ultimate understanding and ultimate peace. This follows the example of Buddha himself, also known as Siddhartha Gautama. Of course, enlightenment is a lofty goal that you can pursue if you are so inclined, but the goal of this book is to put you on the path toward worldly mindfulness. So, if you do not have the time to ponder the mysteries of the universe, have no fear! We will simply journey toward personal peace rather than universal peace. This will be the aim of our dharmic practice, and you can begin to consider how this philosophy of harmony connects to your relationship with food.

It should be noted that mindfulness does not require you to adopt a foreign religion in order for it to be successful. Rather, eastern religion and eastern philosophy are closely intermingled and often considered one and the same, and while practices derived from such philosophies—namely, yoga and meditation—draw strongly from these religious foundations, they are considered the physical manifestations of the philosophy, so there is no need to dwell too long on the distinctly religious elements of their origins. This is why mindfulness, meditation, and yoga have been so easily adapted into the western mindset; eastern religion has more in common with western philosophies than western religions, and many people even consider eastern religion more accessible and understandable than western philosophy!

Knowing the complete history of mindfulness is not required in order to start practicing simple mindfulness techniques today. However, being aware of its development and the various incarnations it has in different religious practices can help you better understand what types of mindfulness philosophies and techniques are best suited to your lifestyle. Do you wish to dedicate yourself to the ancient mindfulness teachings of Hinduism, or do you seek enlightenment by way of the Buddhist sati? Depending on what form of mindfulness works best for you, your path toward a healthy eating mindset can vary greatly from another. This is because each person will take their own unique approach toward mindfulness, and learning mindfulness with respect to different traditions can further differentiate your mindful practices in ways that reflect your needs and goals. No matter what route you choose, it is sure to help instruct you on your journey toward a healthy eating mindset!

The Mind-Body Connection

Western medicine has acknowledged the strong connection between physical health and the mind's perception of the body for centuries. In the early nineteenth century, doctors used placebos to make patients feel better—even though the placebo "medicine" did not actually have an effect on their physical health. In addition, psychosomatic illnesses—that is, sicknesses or injuries created by or intensified by the mind—have been shown to have very real effects on the physical body, meaning that issues originating in the mind can be directly translated to physical complications under the correct circumstances. In order to address this, the interdisciplinary medical field of psychosomatic medicine has been developed to seriously explore the way that psychological, social, and behavioral factors affect bodily processes and overall health. Through psychosomatic medicine, psychotherapy has been integrated into traditional medical techniques to treat physical illnesses and injuries believed to have a mental component. This demonstrates that the mind can not only generate physical discomfort or pain but that it can also heal physical issues. In this light, we can approach the mind-body connection as a way to improve our overall physical health by taking a mental approach.

In order to understand mindfulness' impact on your holistic health, consider the example of yoga. In yoga, mindfulness techniques are used to keep your focus in the present while addressing the needs and limitations of your body. For example, the "body scan" used in yogic practices is similar to the act of creating awareness of the body in mindfulness practices. Often, yogis or meditators begin by taking a mindful inventory of their physical self, sometimes starting at the feet and working their way up to the tip of their head, or vice versa. The body scan is designed to bring awareness to any stiffness, aches, or other issues in the body while celebrating the areas where you feel healthy and limber. While going forth with this knowledge, an individual is ideally able to move in a way that best addresses their physical needs on that day.

This ability to acknowledge your limits and address your needs has been incorporated into positive psychology due to its effectiveness in helping patients understand how they can live in a way that improves their condition without pushing them beyond their emotional boundaries. Some of the major benefits of mindfulness practice alongside traditional psychological methods are the reduction of stress, the treatment of depression and negative thoughts, and increasing general well-being. The adoption of eastern practices into western medicine is a relatively recent development, and whereas fifty years ago doctors may have relied on prescription pills to treat a patient, they now are able to teach patients mindfulness techniques so that they may engage in healing themselves from the inside out. This mirrors the way that a healthy eating mindset will guide you toward improving your relationship with food in an active and positive way, as opposed to the traditional route of diets, detoxes, and weight-loss pills, which do nothing for your mental well-being.

How and why mindfulness techniques are effective: To a cynic, the benefits of mindfulness over traditional dieting methods may still be doubtful. In order to dispel such doubts, consider the flexibility of mindfulness techniques. First, mindfulness can be practiced anywhere and at any time. Whereas a diet plan limits you to eating at certain times (and eating only certain foods), a healthy eating mindset allows you to acknowledge your cravings and consider the best way to address them. Perhaps you are on a subway and see an advertisement for a delicious-looking burger. If you are on a strict diet, you may become frustrated with your inability to eat what you are craving. To a person practicing mindfulness, however, it is simple to acknowledge that the advertisement accomplished its objective of making you desire the product. You can then consider your options: you can go out and buy that burger, or you can seek out a similar, yet healthier alternative, perhaps even making it yourself. Even if there is no inciting incident, you can regularly remind yourself of your goals and the way you wish to achieve them. Mindful eating allows you to acknowledge your hunger and understand that such desires are completely natural—you can then determine if you are truly hungry or if your mind is causing you to feel that way because you are bored, upset, or influenced by something outside of you. Mindfulness is also extremely versatile; you can adopt any number of practices to best suit your lifestyle needs. On the other hand, most traditional diet plans are extremely limited and prescriptive, dictating what you can and cannot do. In contrast, mindfulness encourages you to personalize your practice to fit your schedule, your physical needs, and your emotional desires.

Mindful eating practices encourage harmony among your body, conscious mind, and subconscious desires. This addresses all three as part of a whole: you. In understanding this, you can remind yourself that all of your subconscious desires proceed from your physical needs and your mental influences. Just as your stomach is a part of your body, your desires are a part of your physical and mental self. With this knowledge, we can approach mindfulness not as a way of eradicating your desires but as a way of appreciating them as manifestations of your physical and emotional needs so that you can better control and direct them. This allows you to harness the potentially negative energy of subconscious desires into a positive force in order to better understand yourself. Once you are able to separate your subconscious desires from your present physical and emotional needs—while also understanding that they interact within the greater whole of you as an individual—you will be able to achieve complete awareness over the physical and mental spheres of your relationship with the world, including your relationship with food.

Creating Awareness

By creating awareness through mindfulness practice, you gain a deeper understanding of both your body and your mind. Rather than trying to ignore or avoid problems you may have, mindfulness encourages you to face those problems so that you can decide how to solve them. Scientists have found that by simply creating awareness through mindfulness, you can reduce and relieve your stress levels, decrease the risk of heart disease, lower your blood pressure, alleviate chronic aches and pains, improve the quality of your sleep, and reduce gastrointestinal issues. All of these wonderful benefits are tied to the mere practice of being aware of your body and mind! If you wish to experience these benefits alongside developing a healthy relationship with food, then you no doubt want to begin your mindfulness practice right away. Creating awareness of your physical body is the first step that many people take on their mindfulness journey, so it is best advised to follow in their footsteps in order to see the best results. As mentioned above, the body scan is a simple and effective way to start your mindfulness practice and increase awareness of your physical needs. Be sure to take your time and address every part of your body. Do you feel stiff today? Try to locate the source of that stiffness, starting with a region of the body— midsection, extremities, etc.—and then narrow down until you can pinpoint the exact source. Then ask yourself what you can do to alleviate that stiffness and relax your body. Perhaps engage in some mindful stretching, being careful not to overexert yourself. Work your entire body while focusing on the source of stiffness in order to get the most out of your mindfully guided physical practice.

You can also engage directly with mental awareness in order to guide future physical practices. Meditation is an ancient and widely practiced technique that allows you to address your mental needs, like a body scan for your mind. You can start with a simple five-minute meditation if you are unfamiliar with the practice, and then slowly work your way up to ten-minute, fifteen-minute, and longer meditations. Many experts suggest daily practice of ten minutes every morning, but you can tailor the practice to fit your lifestyle and present needs best. Begin by finding a comfortable seat, relaxing your eyes, and breathing slowly and deeply. Try to focus on how you feel in the present moment, perhaps noticing if you feel tired or stressed, and then asking yourself why you feel that way. Do not dwell on the negative emotions that may accompany the sources of your discomfort, but instead acknowledge them and then send them out of your mind. Once you have addressed any mental issue, you may be experiencing that day, ask yourself how you can fix those issues. Similar to stretching an aching joint, attempt to "exercise" your mind to vanquish negative thoughts and feelings. For example, if you are feeling sad today, remind yourself of everything that you have to be joyful about, such as the simple blessings that you have in your life. If you are feeling stressed, remind yourself that there are certain things that you have no control over, and your only duty is to do what you can in the time that you have been given. Create perspective in your mental space—how big is a problem in comparison with all the goodness that you have in your life? If you find your thoughts wandering to something else, like memories of a movie you saw last night, quietly refocus yourself and take comfort in knowing that everyone's mind wanders sometimes. Just breathe deeply and try to find a relaxing space to exist within. When you feel that you have accomplished a small gain in awareness, you can slowly come back into the physical present. As you leave your practice for the day, try to take that feeling of peace and awareness with you throughout the rest of your actions.

Applying mindfulness techniques to healthy eating: These simple practices can help you find awareness in your daily activities, including eating. Remind yourself to always be present in your actions, creating awareness of what you are eating, as well as when you feel the need to eat. This will prevent you from mindlessly snacking and suddenly thinking: I did not realize I ate that much! Instead, being aware and present in all your actions will allow you to question what you are eating and why. For example, when offered food, do you eat it because you are hungry or because you feel the need to accept a "gift" in such a social situation? By thinking about your subconscious motivations for eating, you will be able to gain clarity on your eating habits and slowly transform them into healthier choices. Whenever faced with a choice involving food, always ask yourself how you can act in a way that will benefit your physical and mental health. Learn to decline food politely—perhaps you can even explain your motivations and be open and vulnerable, as mentioned in Chapter One! Also, take time to evaluate your choices. An important tenet in mindful practice is the act of slowing down and meditating on every action. Instead of rushing through life without thinking about all of your choices, take a deep breath, and fully consider every action that you take. This will create awareness of your circumstances, choice, and the effects of your actions. The understanding that you gain from awareness will help guide you to the best action to take, therefore reshaping your old eating habits into a new healthy eating mindset!

Why you feel the need to eat: The most important aspect of mindfulness in relation to eating is the understanding of your body's relationship to food. Everyone knows that people need food to survive, but food plays many other roles in our lives in addition to being a mere source of nutrients. As we have discussed, sharing meals is a powerful social symbol throughout human history. In the past, hunting was not only a method of providing meat for families but also a popular sport and pastime. Likewise, gardening, farming, and harvesting are often family or community efforts, and harvest festivals have celebrated this relationship between communities and food production for centuries. Unique regional food is also central to many cultures, and traditional recipes and meals are often identified as synonymous with some cultures. In addition, food comforts people and is sometimes considered medicine for the soul. Look no further than the popularity of chicken soup as comfort food or the prevalence of "soul food" in the southern United States. It is obvious that food is much more important to human beings than just being simply a source of vitamins and minerals. People eat when they are sad, stressed, bored, or in the company of others who are eating. This emotional and community-influenced aspect of eating is a powerful influence on all people, and sometimes this influence can become overwhelming, resulting in constant hunger, overeating, strange cravings, and a generally unhealthy and negative relationship with food. Everything about our psyche as humans and about our physical existence tells us that we need to eat, and it is common for those influences to overwhelm us, especially in the age of instant gratification. Mindfulness asks us to acknowledge all these factors as influencing us in sometimes unrecognized ways. As a result, we may feel the need to eat and not understand why without meditating on our influences. Creating awareness of these influences and slowing down in order to address our needs and options allows us to curb unhealthy eating choices while developing new, healthy habits.

It can be difficult to catalog and question each desire at the beginning—but as you become more familiar with your body and mind, you will learn to quickly and easily interpret the many influences and desires that affect your eating habits. Be sure to regularly practice your mindfulness techniques such as body scans and meditation in order to establish this awareness and reduce and eradicate unhealthy habits, and then you can move on to creating an active aspect of your healthy eating mindset in order to encourage the growth of new healthy eating habits. This active portion of your healthy mindset will help you to make major lifestyle changes, such as adapting to a new diet plan, while providing you with the tools you need to sustain your healthy eating journey and propel you forwards. We will discuss these active mindfulness techniques and outline how to implement them in the next chapter.

CHAPTER 3: CREATING YOUR HEALTHY MINDSET

Now that you have a basic understanding of the practice of awareness, you can begin to develop new habits through what is termed active mindfulness practices. Active practices do not replace the awareness-building practices of body scans and regular meditation that we discussed in the previous chapter, but they instead act in tandem with awareness-building so that they complement and strengthen one another. You may even find yourself able to perform the two practices simultaneously! That is to say, while awareness accounts for the flow and direction of your current energy state, active practices redirect that energy and channel it into new modes of healthy expression. For example, during a moving meditation (a meditative session that involves taking different yoga postures to increase awareness), you may discover that you are under a lot of pressure and feel emotional pressure manifesting in stiff shoulders. Using this awareness, you can move to a posture that releases built-up stress from your shoulders, thereby recognizing your current energy flow and then redirecting it to improve your mental and physical health that day.

There are many different kinds of active practices, ranging from activities that directly align with awareness-building, such as moving meditation and yoga—to activities that prioritize physical health, such as general exercise. In this chapter, we will discuss two important active practices that directly impact your healthy eating mindset, meal tracking and flexible diet plans, and how they improve your body's relationship with food. As you learn about these active practices, keep in mind the image of diverging paths and the idea of your destination. This will guide you as you decide which aspects of these practices you choose to adopt and how you personalize these practices to best benefit your lifestyle changes.

Keeping a Food Diary

One active practice that is extremely effective in continuing to build awareness while developing new healthy eating habits is tracking what you eat. Keeping a food diary is a widely practiced method of both weight loss and nutritious and mindful eating because it forces you to record everything that you eat so that you can later reflect on your choices and consider whether or not you are living your healthiest life. There are many different ways to track what you eat, and there are even phone apps designed specifically for this purpose! If you want to go the old-school way, though, you open yourself up to limitless options of personalization and growth in your practice. Many people opt to use a simple notebook as their food diary, and this is beneficial because you can choose a notebook with a fun cover to best encourage you to carry it around and use it regularly. In setting up your food diary, you can approach it in one of two ways: as a traditional diary with paragraph-style entry logs, or as a more technical tracker with charts where you can record your meals and snacks. Some people like to be very detailed with their food diaries, recording their caloric intake, and calculating the nutrients they consumed. If this sounds too complicated for your lifestyle, have no fear! Even recording a description of what you ate, such as "a pizza slice and a glass of water," can help you visualize your habits. Take a few days to discover what works best for you, and then try to stick to the practice once you have settled on a certain style. After a while, you should be able to look back at your old entries and view your food diary as a description of your growth and progress.

If you would like a simple template to adapt into your own customized meal tracker, feel free to begin from the following example:

Date: Monday, August 19, 2019			
Food/Drink	Time	Servings	Calories
Pizza	12:00 pm	1	285
Soda	12:00 pm	1	150
Daily Totals:			435

One benefit of keeping a more detailed food diary is that it allows you to track your caloric intake, which experts say encourages you to consume fewer calories. Although calories are not unhealthy in and of themselves, excessive consumption of more calories than your body requires causes those calories—which are units of the amount of energy stored in food that is needed to raise the temperature of one gram of water by one degree Celsius—to build up, and your body then stores them as fat. The average adult woman burns approximately 2,000 calories a day, so nutritionists generally recommend that you should consume 2,000 calories a day to replenish your energy. However, since most people do not concern themselves with tracking their daily intake of calories, they often run the risk of overconsuming and subsequently gain weight due to the excessive amounts of calories they store. Calorie counting itself sometimes comes with negative connotations, but this is only in reference to traditional dieting plans. With mindful eating, we seek to replace empty calories with healthy alternatives found in other foods like fruits and vegetables. Because keeping a food diary allows you to make the connection between calorie amounts and types of food, people who track their meals are more like to make healthy and mindful choices. The practice of recording and evaluating your portion sizes and the number of servings has a very similar benefit (we will further discuss servings sizes and portions in Chapter 5: Curbing Overeating and How to Feel Full). Studies actually suggest that people who keep food diaries are likely to lose and keep off twice as much weight as those who do not. Furthermore, by recording when you are eating, you can better understand your body's cravings and how to address them in healthy ways. This is because your record-keeping will alert you to periods of snacking or binging, making you more aware of issues you may have with sticking to a healthy diet. It can also show you unhealthy patterns of eating, such as not eating during the day and then overeating at night. In this way, tracking your meals helps you consciously make better, healthier choices while also normalizing the structure of your eating habits.

Non-Restrictive Diet Plans

As discussed in the first chapter, there are several non-restrictive diet plans that you can use to supplement your healthy eating mindset. It is important to emphasize the difference between these non-restrictive diet plans and traditional short-term diets. The goal is to alter what foods make you feel happy and healthful while eating rather than limit you to what you feel like you have to eat. Not only is this dieting mindset more forgiving for your mind and body, but it is also more effective in the long run. Researchers at UCLA have conducted long-term studies on the effectiveness of traditional dieting and found that although participants saw a five to ten percent decrease in overall body weight during the height of their dieting, once the diet period ended, they put the weight back on. This shows that dieting is at most a short-term solution for changing your physical health, whereas diet plans focus on long-term improvement in both the body and the mind. As mentioned before, the way that traditional diets are structured focuses on depriving the body of something it wants, like ice cream or potato chips. This mindset of deprivation can lead to malnutrition and anorexia when taken to the extreme. In contrast, a healthy eating diet plan asks you to reconsider your eating habits and find ways to replace unhealthy snacks with something healthier. This way, rather than cutting out a large portion of your old diet, you exchange one thing for another. The core of healthy eating diet plans is making healthy choices rather than excluding food from your diet.

The three basic diet plan options outlined in Chapter One—organic, vegetarian/vegan, and garden-to-table—should be taken as suggestions of ways to reshape your current diet. Here, it is important to define the term "diet" as something that does not refer to a restrictive plan that dictated what you can and cannot eat but as your actual present pattern of consumption. This is the key to creating an image of a healthy diet in your mind: rather than limit yourself to what sounds healthy in general, try to take into consideration what your mind and body need and how you can best meet those needs. This mode of thinking will allow you to alter your current diet to include healthier options, and once you become accustomed to those new options, you will find it easy to simply leave behind your old bad habits of eating unhealthy foods. The organic option actively encourages you to seek out all-natural alternatives to food that you already eat. Many stores stock organic versions of all your favorite meals and snacks. The vegetarian or vegan diet helps you exchange unhealthy animal-based foods with delicious plant-based options. Likewise, the garden-to-table plan guides you in seeking local, natural replacements for the highly processed foods that you were familiar with eating. In this way, a healthy diet plan actively helps you reprogram your body's hunger while curtailing unhealthy desires in your mind. However, it is important to remember that these diets by themselves will not be enough to create and maintain a healthy eating mindset. It is important that you continue to practice awareness and use other mindfulness techniques in addition to adjusting our diet. This creates an emotional backup to your physical actions, establishing that positive feedback loop we mentioned earlier. If you do not maintain your mindfulness throughout your journey, you may find yourself becoming disillusioned with your diet plan and abandoning the practice. That is why you must envision our journey as perpetual rather than short-term and limited. In a sense, the healthy eating mindset journey is very similar to the Buddhist's quest for enlightenment, since perfection always seems out of reach. This constant yearning and eternal personal improvement are cyclical rather than linear, and we should rationalize our journey accordingly.

Allowing your diet plan to evolve: As your healthy eating mindset evolves, you may find that you must incorporate certain foods that are outside of your current diet plan or that you desire to change your diet plan completely. This is perfectly normal and should be encouraged, as healthy eating exists in many forms, and there is not a singular correct way to be healthy.

This is another key distinguishing aspect between healthy eating diet plans and traditional dieting—the flexibility and growth afforded within the healthy eating mindset allows you to personalize and alter your diet plan according to your unique needs. This flexibility is forgiving, whereas traditional diet plans frame change either as "failure" or "completion." As we have learned so far, slip-ups are human and should not be equated with failure, whereas the achievement of short-term goals does not necessarily guarantee success in the long run—only persistence and dedication will lead you to your desired end goal, which is actually the journey in and of itself. The healthy eating mindset diet plans encourage growth and learning rather than focusing on weight loss on its own; we must understand that weight loss is only a small part of achieving a healthier life overall.

Learning to Appreciate Your Body's Relationship with Food

As we have discussed, your body seeks food first and foremost as a source of nourishment for a healthy life. But there is more beyond the need to eat to survive. Everyone has unique needs according to their body. If you are an athlete, you must consume more calories so that you can have enough energy to exercise and perform your athletic feats; diabetics need to regulate the glucose in their blood, and so they must balance their sugar intake or receive insulin shots. Likewise, every person in the world has unique needs in relation to food, and part of your journey will be discovering those needs. You may find that you require more caffeine than your friends, for instance. These needs should not be dismissed as problems to be solved but rather as part of your body's relationship with food. Recall from the last chapter that your desires are as much a part of you as your stomach. Just because you cannot see it does not mean that it is not just as present in your life.

One of the biggest hurdles to appreciating your body's relationship with food is a negative body image. Unfortunately, in today's society, so much emphasis and value are placed on the way a person looks.

Usually, the people who are hurt the most by this are people who are considered overweight. If you are overweight or have a highly negative self-image of your body, you likely have an unhealthy relationship with food. The purpose of the healthy eating mindset is to address this relationship first and foremost. That is why, in addition to the mindfulness techniques given in this book to encourage healthy eating habits, we should also address ways of improving body image. The first method of improving body image is to verbalize what you love about yourself. This can help you identify new ways to express self-love and discover beautiful aspects of your physical body that you can use to improve your body image. Psychologists suggest leaving notes for yourself around the house, especially near mirrors, so that you can regularly remind yourself that you are beautiful and that you are loved. Try to compliment a different part of yourself every day to ensure that you are giving attention to all of your body—do not let insecurities stamp out appreciation for yourself. Also, try to eliminate negative thoughts and words concerning your body or other people's bodies. If you have negative thoughts about yourself, like criticisms of your weight, clothes, or hair, try to silence those thoughts and replace them with positive thoughts. Likewise, do not allow unfair criticisms of others' appearances to persist in your life, because the way we see others sometimes reflects the way we see ourselves. Getting rid of negativity across the board is the best way to see an instant improvement in your life.

In addition, you may benefit from limiting your media consumption. First, unrealistic representations and expectations of human bodies run rampant in movies, television, and social media. Second, online comments can be excessively cruel, and cyberbullying should never be taken lightly. Just as negative comments about other people in real life can have an equally negative effect on your, mean comments about someone's body online can be detrimental to your mental health, especially if you identify with the person (usually a celebrity) being criticized. To capitalize off of all the hard work you have done to nurture self-love, consider directly confronting your body image issues by talking to a therapist or seeking out resources to help you improve your body image.

When you are comfortable with your body, you will be comfortable with your body's relationship with food. Allow yourself to relax while eating, letting go of the emotional or social anxieties surrounding food. When you are truly relaxed with the act of eating, you will be at peace physically so that you can eat in order to meet your body's needs, mentally so that you can appreciate the delicious qualities of the food and its sources, and socially so that you can eat with others without feeling pressure to eat less or more. Relaxed eating is directly connected to self-love because it draws on trust that you are benefiting your health and the comfort of knowing that you are performing an act of autonomous self-expression rather than feeling restrained or pressured. Furthermore, a healthy relationship with food will encourage flexibility. Whereas a strict diet plan will damage your relationship with food and make you feel like you have to eat specific foods in specific amounts, the healthy eating mindset positively develops your body's relationship with food by encouraging experimentation and personalization. This flexibility allows for forgiveness and understanding if you have a sudden unquenchable craving for a snack that is less healthy than what you think you should be eating. Having potato chips every once in a while will not kill you, and the mindset connected to a healthy relationship with food knows this. When you develop a healthy understanding of your body's relationship with food, you will be able to accept moments like these while still aiming for a consistently healthy diet. Finally, you will be able to understand and appreciate your body's need for a balanced diet. This means that you will see the error in diets that require you to eat a single type of food and nothing else, and you will also recognize the importance of experimentation when it comes to your own diet. Of course, you need to get all of your required nutrients to be healthy, which means eating your fruits and vegetables, but what else can a balanced diet look like? You can try diets that include everything in moderation, or you can experiment with wildly varying types of foods and explore your options. In this way, balance can be closely linked to flexibility in that it encourages healthy variety.

Everyone has a different relationship with food—and understanding this is the first step that you can take in developing your healthy mindset. Depending on what kind of relationship you had with food prior to embarking on this journey, you may start at a different position than someone else. This may require you to focus on rebuilding your relationship with food extensively—as is in the case with some people with negative body image issues—or you may simply have to restructure your relationship to prioritize a mindset of growth. Either way, understanding the techniques of mindfulness and how they can improve your understanding of the role that food plays in your overall health is vital. With this in mind, you should use your food diary and your diet plan in order to better appreciate your body's relationship with food and discover ways that you can improve that relationship. Learn to look for improvement in small ways and reward yourself accordingly when you feel that you have made progress, such as indulging in chocolate, some ice cream, or another food that other diets may force you to give up. Understand that growth is cyclical rather than linear because you are constantly redefining your baseline and moving your goal further. Rationalize this growth by focusing on the small actions that you take in the present and how those may relate to the overall growth and improvement that you wish to see. Take the time to refamiliarize yourself with your patterns of consumption and how your diet can address those patterns in healthy and mindful ways.

CHAPTER 4: EATING YOUR FEELINGS?

Mindfulness brings awareness to your actions, which is why it is super-effective in curbing overeating. Oftentimes, overeating corresponds with your emotional states—usually the negative ones. This is where mindfulness really gets a chance to shine, as it has been proven by many psychologists to be effective in treating negative thoughts and feelings. The treatment of these negative emotions rather than the attempt to cover them up not only makes you feel better in the present but also prevents you from overeating, which could potentially harm you emotionally in the future. Emotional eating must be taken seriously and addressed as a very real hurdle in your journey toward a healthy eating mindset. Just because you feel secure in your emotions does not mean that you are immune to bouts of emotional eating.

Emotional eating is actually one of the major reasons that popular traditional diets fail—once you become frustrated with a diet, your daily emotional pains may become exaggerated, thus causing you to seek physical and emotional comfort in food. Eating can be used as a way of relieving stress, coping with unpleasant emotions, or rewarding yourself. In this way, eating can quickly become an unhealthy coping mechanism, and you can fall into the unhealthy pattern of indulging in overeating habits. Although eating may temporarily assuage your negative emotions, the causes of those feelings remain unaddressed, and they will likely return—thus leaving you frustrated or guilty with your initial reaction of eating your feelings. In order to prevent emotional eating while you work towards developing a healthy eating mindset, it is important to acknowledge the major causes of emotional overeating and understand your mind's relationship with food. Once you are equipped with this knowledge, you can begin taking measure to curb emotional eating and channel your energy into more productive ways to address your negative emotions.

Major Causes of Overeating

Many people find themselves mindlessly snacking all the time, be it at home, at a bar, or at a friend's house. Since eating can be very social in nature, others' eating habits often affect yours in unhealthy ways. This mindless consumption is one such way. Eating when you do not need to eat and without paying attention is one of the major causes of overeating. Another major cause of overeating finds its roots in your emotional states. Most people are familiar with the phrase "eating your feelings." This idiom has a very real source in psychology; referring back to our discussion of comfort food, many people associate the act of eating with warm feelings of comfort, fulfillment, and calmness. Therefore, the act of eating when sad or hurt is meant to make you feel better from the inside out. Although food can be a very effective emotional medicine, it must be moderated and balanced, just like chemical prescriptions.

Emotional hunger is distinct from physical hunger. Whereas physical hunger builds through longer gaps between meals, emotional hunger may hit suddenly and powerfully due to an emotional trigger. This emotional hunger may feel even more potent than physical hunger, causing you to crave specific types of food with a surprising sense of urgency. The type of food that you crave is your preferred type of comfort food, and it may seem like the only thing that can satisfy your craving. Although healthy and green foods would physically fill you up, your emotions may tell you that only a burger or potato chips will truly end your craving. Likewise, physical hunger usually tells your body that it needs a certain amount of nourishment, which leads to feeling full, but emotional hunger often leads to overeating, even to the point where you have eaten too much and now feel uncomfortable or sick to your stomach. This is a major sign of an unhealthy coping mechanism since it often makes you feel worse than you initially did. On top of this, emotional hunger is difficult to satisfy—so even when you overeat, your cravings may not disappear. This is because physical hunger originates in the stomach, while emotional hunger is located in your mind. Emotion hunger is triggered by emotions and then fed by mental images of your favorite foods. However, those mental cravings do not always correspond to physical realities, which is why the cravings are difficult, if not impossible, to satisfy. To make matters worse, while the act of emotional overeating falsely promises to alleviate negative thoughts and feelings and in turn may create new physical issues, it also often leads to compounded negative emotions; emotional overeating often creates feelings of guilt, shame, and regret.

This is why emotional eating must be considered at

the beginning of your healthy eating mindset journey rather than being overlooked. It can be detrimental to your health and your confidence in the healthy eating mindset plan, so be sure not to trivialize its causes and negative effects. Training yourself to avoid emotional eating takes time, but the awareness that you can cultivate through mindfulness can quickly help you identify emotional eating urges. From there, you will be able to take preventative measures and learn to cope with your emotional eating urges in healthy ways. However, if you find yourself still falling prey to the emotional eating trap, be sure to forgive yourself and put your actions in perspective—although you are training your mind to develop new, healthy relationships with food, there are certain triggers that are highly difficult to address, such as high-stress levels.

A Closer Look at Emotional Stress Eating

Emotional stress eating is one of the more difficult types of emotional eating to address. This is because stress cravings exist not only in the mind's mental images, but also manifest themselves very physically in the body. Chronic stress runs rampant in today's fast-paced world, and the negative effects of chronic stress can appear in all aspects of your life, including your diet. Short-term bursts of stress, also known as acute stress episodes, can reduce your appetite to the point of stomach-twisting nervousness due to the production of adrenaline, but long-term or chronic stress produces a different hormone that actually intensifies your hunger. Chronic stress causes the release of the cortisol, which increases your appetite and may make you more energized in general; typically, cortisol levels should return to normal after a period of time, but chronic stress causes your cortisol levels to remain elevated. This is a major problem since cortisol production creates cravings for foods high in fat content, sugar, or both. This is because fatty and sugary foods act as negative feedback to stress and dampen its effects. However, if you suffer from chronic stress, your stress levels will continue to rise, you will regularly crave large amounts of fat and sugar, and a hellish cycle of stress eating can develop. This is actually quite dangerous because stress has many lasting effects on the mind and body, and it can also cause poor sleep, a lack of motivation to exercise, a desire for increased alcohol intake, and general negative emotions, all of which can contribute to poor overall health, not to mention weight gain.

Emotional stress eating is considered a form of binge eating, which is a pattern of consuming large amounts of food in a single sitting. Patterns of binge eating are actually shown to induce or increase anxiety, which leads to more overall stress. If episodes of binge eating due to stress begin to occur at least once a week for an extended period of time, this pattern is further classified as a binge eating disorder (BED). BED is a serious medical condition that requires the help of a medical professional because generally, people who suffer from BED show a complete lack of control of overeating and an impaired ability to regulate emotional impulses. The development of BED results in a temporarily elevated mood after a binge, which encourages the continuation of the binging pattern and leads to a chronic disorder. Luckily, stress eating does not always lead to the development of BED, especially when addressed early on. This is why you should make efforts to improve your mental and emotional relationship with food at the beginning of your healthy eating mindset journey, even if you have not suffered from stress eating in the past.

Thankfully, there are simple ways to address and ultimately prevent stress eating. By focusing on stress' relationship with food and hunger, you will be able to start small and work your way out into dealing with stress in all parts of your life. As mentioned several times already, a healthy eating mindset encourages you to develop holistic habits of health, which positively affect your life as a whole, even in ways not directly linked to eating. This wonderful connection between mind and body, food and feelings, and health and happiness is not immediately apparent to some people. That is why, if you find yourself positively impacted by this book, you are encouraged to share your experience with fellow readers by leaving a review on Amazon for this book. The lovely nature of mindfulness is that it helps you visualize ways to not only help yourself but also help others. As you continue to increase your awareness of yourself within the larger network of life in the world, return regularly to your thoughts, feelings, and emotions in order to ground yourself in the practice of mindfulness.

Adapting Your Mindset to Account for Your Emotions

Emotions are the most human aspect of life; they connect us with each other and define our memories, personalities, and experiences of the world. When they get out of control, however, we must carefully call them back into order and remind ourselves that we must rule our emotions rather than letting them rule us. Bringing awareness to both the body and mind can aid you in this endeavor, allowing you to understand better where your emotions come from and how to channel them into healthy actions successfully. For instance, now that we have discussed the causes of emotional stress eating, you can identify such urges when they occur in your life and learn how to best deal with your cravings in a healthy way, such as overcoming the desire to eat sugary and fatty foods. Instead, you can help your body heal from the stress by eating foods high in nutrients like antioxidants, which have been shown to significantly decrease chronic stress levels in a healthy way by improving your immune system's ability to function in stressful situations and supplying your body with a healthy and reliable supply of energy. So while your body might crave ice cream or potato chips, you can acknowledge that these cravings are produced by stress and that, while the food you desire may temporarily relieve you stress cravings, this kind of food will not relieve your stress in the long run and may actually cause more problems for you physically and emotionally. Rather than giving in to these cravings, try to snack on healthy alternatives like almonds, fresh blueberries, avocado, and even limited amounts of dark chocolate. You can also prepare meals that anticipate spikes in stress levels and contain nutrients that will help keep cortisol levels down, as well as experiment with home-cooked meals of grass-fed beef, roasted asparagus, salmon, and other foods rich in antioxidants.

Furthermore, you can use the mindfulness techniques already outlined (body scans, meditation, exercise, food diaries, and diet plans) to help you better understand and control your emotions. Remember that your emotions are a part of you and arise from physical and mental triggers. This means that you should look to understand and control your emotions rather than smother or ignore them. As we have discussed, the first step to mindfully addressing any issue is developing awareness. In addition to the mindfulness techniques above, simply remember to accept your emotions, whether you are feeling sad, angry, guilty, scared, or worried. Acknowledge the causes of your emotions and do not attempt to ignore them—this will only cause your negative emotions to build up until they boil over at a later time. Even if it feels uncomfortable or scary to confront your emotions, the more time you take to be present and aware of your emotions, the easier it will become. Be sure to listen to your emotions because they can usually reveal a hidden element of your conscious mind. For instance, if you feel irrationally angry about something your friend accomplished, it may be due to underlying feelings of inadequacy about performing at the same level. In this way, although you should listen to your emotions, the mindful course of action is distinct from simply allowing your emotions to control you; you should aim to confront your emotions in a constructive manner so that you can heal yourself from within while also learning more about yourself. Once you have become adequately aware of your emotions, take it a step further by trying to identify specific emotional urges. From the example above, you may initially think you are angry—but upon further inspection, you may find that the emotion is actually jealousy or self-consciousness. By specifically addressing these emotions and saying, "I feel angry. I feel jealous. I feel scared," you can not only better understand your feelings but also empower yourself in the understanding that your emotions are part of you. You are neither reduced to your emotions, nor are you controlled by them. By taking identifying and confronting your emotions, you will be able to stay in the present, therefore staying cognizant of the choices in front of you so that you can take healthy and well-informed action. It is only by remaining focus on the present—not dwelling in the past or being unnecessarily worried about the future—that you can make the best choices. Staying aware of your actions in the present will prevent you from doing things that you will regret later, like eating that entire pint of ice cream! Meanwhile, be sure that you positively accept your reactions so that you can build compassion for yourself. This positive reinforcement will satisfy your need for comfort, eliminating the urge to comfort yourself through eating.

The reason that self-compassion is more effective

than comfort food is that internal issues require internal remedies, and physical comforts like food will only have a physical effect, leaving your emotional troubles unaddressed. As you become more acquainted with the practice of self-compassion, it will become second-nature for you to comfort yourself when overpowered with negative emotions. This experience will help you quickly soothe yourself and dispel your negative feelings, leaving room for you to plan a constructive course of action while building new, positive emotions. This will, in turn, help you to realize that your negative emotions are short-lived; although it may feel in the moment that your sadness, anger, or fear is seeping into every aspect of your life and permanently changing your character, you must be able to realize that these feelings are fleeting and come and go according to your situation and mood. This is another reason why being aware and staying in the present is vital to successful mindfulness techniques— knowing that your emotions belong to a moment rather than eternity will provide you with a better perspective on your situation and inform your actions in positive and constructive ways. Many times, your negative emotions will not even require immediate action or reaction. Instead, you can use your awareness of the present to take a step back and simply observe your emotions. Sometimes, your negative feelings will simply evolve and evaporate on their own once you have detached yourself from them. The knowledge that sometimes you can just let your emotions run their course in a passive yet healthy way will be a powerful tool in your arsenal of mindfulness techniques. Once your emotions are dealt with—either by taking mindful action or allowing the emotions to wind down on their own—you can further investigate their sources and how they affect you. Take time to ask yourself if your negative emotions are part of a repeating pattern and, if so, how you can deal with that pattern. Utilize some of the following guided questions to understand your emotions better:

- What triggered my negative emotions?

- What emotions did I experience, and how did they develop?

- Did my emotions draw mostly off of my internal thoughts or the actions of someone else?

- What thoughts came into my mind while experiencing these emotions? Did I mostly think of the present, past, or future?

- How can I address the cause of my emotions and perhaps prevent them from occurring/reduce their severity in future instances?

These questions will not only help you better understand the emotional episode that you just experienced, but they will also equip you to better deal with future episodes. Allowing yourself to observe and question your emotions helps to separate your rational, thinking mind from your emotional responses, which will help you better understand what appropriate actions you can take to address and assuage your negative emotions in the future. By preparing yourself to confront your emotions healthily, you reduce the chances of falling back into unhealthy coping mechanisms like emotional eating. In this way, mindfulness not only helps you better understand your feelings, but it also helps you to avoid negative reactions to those feelings.

In addition to these awareness-creating and preventative mindfulness techniques, you can also incorporate healthy actions into the process of dealing with negative emotions. First, consult your food diary and consider changing the timing of your meals and snacks to coincide with periods of stress eating. This is helpful because you will be less likely to crave food if you already have a relatively full stomach. So if you feel more stressed in the early evening, consider having a later lunch to help prevent your stress from developing into emotional hunger. In addition, you can prepare small healthy snacks like veggie sticks so that you can reach for a healthy alternative if you do feel overcome with emotional hunger. Be sure to limit your snacking though—even with healthy snacks, stress cravings can make you go overboard with any food, as suggested by the common phrase, "too much of a good thing." With this in mind, be sure to keep your snacks to a single serving size when preparing for possible emotional episodes. You can also try to engage in activities that will take your mind off of eating or even distract you from your stressors. This is different from ignoring your emotions, as you are redirecting your emotional energy to a different activity rather than attempting to bottle up that negative outburst. You can work off some of your stress by exercising, talking to a friend about your emotions, or engaging in a favorite hobby of yours. You can also try to directly address and reduce your negative emotions by meditating or doing some yoga.

If you do not confront your emotions during the activity, be sure to do so afterward so that you can turn the emotional episode into a learning moment. If you experience stress while performing a specific activity and feel that you cannot take a break, either because of a deadline or other responsibility that you must meet, consider approaching the activity itself in the same way that we addressed negative emotions. Rationalize the activity in your mind and connect it to you how you feel in the present. Be sure to flatly address unhealthy coping mechanisms in such a way: "Stress eating will not help me meet my deadline. In fact, it may even slow me down." Address your emotions and desires in a straightforward way while remaining realistic. Allow yourself to nibble on a healthy snack if your cravings may negatively affect your health and if they cannot be dealt with in another way. The most important element of mindfulness is the process of recognizing your limits, and your mindfulness techniques should never feel uncomfortable or take the form of punishment. In the end, you should be acting in a way that benefits your health first and foremost, even if that means losing a little ground in the moment. Keep in mind that mental health is equally as important as physical health—in fact, the two are often inseparable—and you should not restrict yourself if it causes you any mental distress. It is perfectly acceptable to allow yourself to indulge slightly in emotional eating as long as you limit yourself to a healthy amount and promise to work on eliminating the habit in the future.

All of this is part of a growth mindset—rather than requiring instant change, adopting a mindset of awareness allows you to forgive yourself and work toward improvement at your own pace. In addition, this improvement is not focused on simply eliminating emotional eating but also addressing the causes of emotional eating, which will both improve your physical health and enrich your mental well-being. Emotional eating takes many forms, such as comfort food for when you are sad, angry, or stressed out, and a mindset of awareness accounts for all of these variations. This is because a healthy eating mindset is concerned with your holistic health rather than ineffectively pinpointing one bad habit—it allows you to work on improving your overall health in a way that fosters self-love.

CHAPTER 5: CURBING OVEREATING AND HOW TO FEEL FULL

As discussed in the previous chapter, overeating is often a symptom of a lack of awareness in your life. When you are not alert to what you are consuming (and when), you are at risk of mindlessly overeating. This type of overeating can take the form of a binging episode or manifest as constant snacking throughout the day. Similar to emotional eating, mindless eating attempts to fill some sort of mental need. Oftentimes, people mindlessly eat when they are bored or focused on another passive activity, such as watching television. The double-edged sword of binge-watching and binge-eating is especially dangerous, as the increased calorie intake is not burned at all while you sit on the couch and watch episode after episode of your favorite show.

Hence, how do you prevent yourself from engaging in these unhealthy habits? First, awareness through mindfulness techniques can help reduce the time you spend mindlessly eating while passive. As previously explained, awareness allows you to stay focused on the present and helps inform healthy and productive actions. If you are fully aware of your passive state and the unhealthy aspect of consuming large amounts of foods throughout the day, you will be less likely to engage in such unhealthy habits. You can build awareness every day by using the techniques already mentioned in this book—such as meditation, meal tracking, and developing a healthy diet plan. This will increase your awareness of what you consume, in addition to opening up your ability to be aware of everything in your life, including your relative activity or passivity. Once you are aware of the bad habits you may have, you can work toward curbing these habits and replacing them with new, productive activities, such as watching television while doing easy indoor exercises.

In addition, you can create new, healthy habits to reward yourself for staying mindful of your consumption. If you are a particularly crafty and artistic person, you may wish to embellish your food diary with stickers, illustrations, or ephemera to celebrate your mindful habits. If you find joy in social interaction, you can take to social media to announce your success and consistency in your mindfulness techniques—being cheered on and congratulated by your friends will create positive feedback for your practice. You can also introduce healthy snacks and limited passive activities to your regular schedule. This way, instead of completely cutting out activities like binge-watching from your life, you can limit yourself to a certain amount of time or number of episodes in order to allocate space in your schedule for healthier activities. You can even slowly reduce the time allowed by a little bit every day until you reach a limit that you find acceptable. While doing this, you can switch out your old snacks for new, healthier options. Here are some easy swaps you can make today:

• Instead of buttery, cheesy popcorn, try popcorn flavored with just a hint of sea salt.

• Replace soda or alcoholic beverages with fruit juice, sparkling water, tea, or lemonade.

• Rather than buying regular potato chips, try to stick to baked chips, vegetable chips, or rice cakes.

These alternatives will allow you to continue snacking while watching a movie or television show while providing you with a more nutritious option than your old snack choices. However, be sure to limit yourself to healthy portions and stay aware of your serving sizes. After all, these are meant to be snacks and not meals.

No more mindless eating: In order to successfully curtail mindless eating, keep returning to your mindfulness techniques. Healthier alternatives are a good place to start—but without maintaining your awareness, you are still at risk of overeating. (Yes, you can "overeat" relatively healthy foods!) The only way to completely eradicate mindless eating is to introduce mindfulness into every aspect of your life. By being aware of all your actions as you go through your day, you can avoid mindlessly reaching for a snack. Researchers estimate that the average person makes more than 200 decisions about food every single day, but most people are only aware of a small fraction of those decisions. This explains why mindless eating is such a common problem—many people are subconsciously making decisions about what, when, and how much to eat! Since those decisions are made subconsciously, no rational thought goes into them, and the causes and circumstances from which the choice arose are not examined. This means that subtle advertising can subconsciously influence you to want a soda even if you are not physically thirsty. An outside factor planted that desire in your mind, and then your mind communicates that desire to your body, which generates physical cravings. Before you even think about what made you thirsty or how the sugary beverage may impact your health, you are reaching for a soda! This is how mindless consumption works, and it can be one of the biggest obstacles to a healthy eating mindset. Luckily, there are mindfulness techniques that can make you more aware of your influences and choices, which will prevent you from mindless overeating.

Visual reminders: One of these best ways to combat visual cues that try to influence your subconscious mind is to just turn that technique back on itself. Scientists have determined that many people rely on external influences rather than internal signals when determining if they are hungry, meaning visual reminders can make people either feel hungry or full. This is why seeing a television advertisement of a delicious dinner can make your mouth water even if you just ate. To combat visual cues that make you want to eat more, try to remind yourself that you do not need to eat either by leaving used dishes out for a bit longer after a meal or by putting sticky notes up where you keep your snacks. A simple reminder like "You just ate!" can go a long way in combating mindless eating.

Reorganize your kitchen: Since mindless consumption operates on the basis of not thinking about your food choices, you can disrupt your ability to mindless reach for a snack by simply moving food around in your kitchen and pantry. If you rotate your food storage, you may forget where you put something for a few moments, forcing yourself to think about your actions. Once you start thinking about where you moved the bag of chips, you will remember why you moved the snacks around, thereby alerting yourself to your mindless eating urge. This will likely stop you from overeating! Likewise, if you move all of your favorite snacks to hard to reach places like the top shelf that is just out of reach or back behind all of your canned foods, you may feel inconvenienced enough that you decide it is not worth the trouble. This is doubly effective if you put your healthy options in easy to access places.

Limit your supply: The bottom line is that if you do not have unhealthy foods available, then you cannot eat unhealthy foods! You can work with this knowledge without completely eliminating your access to quick snacks by allowing yourself to empty your supply of a certain food before restocking. By only purchasing one unit of your favorite snack, you limit the amount that you can eat and encourage yourself to "ration" the food. Of course, you can always buy more once you finish the snack, but a limited supply works to discourage overeating at the moment.

Make eating its own activity: Although it can seem unnatural in the current era of multitasking, eating while not using your phone or watching television helps brings awareness to the act of eating. By focusing on eating as its own activity, you eliminate the danger of mindlessly overeating and continuously snacking while distracted by something else. This ability to focus on the act of eating is also related to the practice of slowing down while eating, which we will discuss in Chapter 6: Meditating on Food.

Structured Mealtimes

In addition to using mindfulness techniques to bring awareness to your eating choices, you can also introduce structure to your meals in order to discourage overeating later. Research has shown that having regularly scheduled mealtimes can help train your body only to expect food during designated times. This decreases the occurrence of hunger throughout the day. Skipping meals, fasting, or waiting too long between two meals can cause you to overeat at your next meal, so it is important to make sure you do eat every meal at regular intervals. Researchers at Harvard Medical School have also found that eating regularly scheduled meals can help boost your metabolism. Basically, if you do not eat regular meals, your basal metabolic rate (BMR) decreases, causing you to burn fewer calories and making it easier to gain weight. Another study found that skipping breakfast can actually increase the risk of type 2 diabetes, obesity, and chronic inflammation. This lends credence to the old saying, "Breakfast is the most important meal of the day." Furthermore, eating meals at regular intervals helps keep you energized throughout the day; hunger often corresponds to tiredness, irritability, and fatigue, so it is no surprise that keeping well-fed and well-fueled helps generate more energy.

Another benefit of structured mealtimes is that they help encourage self-control. By staying full throughout the day, courtesy of regular meals, you become less likely to indulge in an unhealthy snack or mindless eating. Studies show that it is easier to maintain an overall healthy diet due to the steady energy provided by regular meals. This includes a lower desire for sugary or fatty foods, less craving for fast food, and an increase in the regular consumption of fruits and vegetables.

Nutritionists also encourage people to eat four or five smaller meals throughout the day rather than three large meals. This is because the practice of eating additional smaller meals coincides better with our natural urges, whereas eating three meals a day is a social construct with no real benefits. If you find yourself craving food between meals and snacking intermittently throughout the day, it is likely that a change in your meal structure will benefit your healthy eating mindset. Once you have transitioned to four or five smaller meals a day, you will be less likely to eat continuously and mindlessly consume snacks. It will also make it easier to not eat between meals since you have a shorter period of time to wait, while also decreasing the probability of overeating at any one meal. By regularly eating smaller meals, you can move away from oversized servings to more manageable amounts of food. This will promote healthy serving sizes, which are also important in a healthy eating mindset.

Smaller Servings

Smaller serving sizes are often the first thing people focus on when trying to lose weight. This is because many people overeat without realizing it. Controlling and limiting your portions will stop you from overeating, so it is no wonder why serving sizes are such a prominent topic among health enthusiasts. The healthy eating mindset also encourages smaller portions, not specifically for the goal of losing weight but because they prevent the unhealthy habit of overeating. Serving sizes are recommended amounts of food for you to consume, which you can then base your portions on. Generally, you should try to limit yourself to portions of a single serving for each food that you eat, because the serving size is based on the amounts of nutrients that the average person eats. You can find the recommended serving size of a particular food at the top of the nutrition label on its packaging, but you can also look up estimates of serving sizes online. It can be very helpful to include serving size information in your food diary, especially if you are looking to decrease your portions while raising your awareness about your diet. The benefits of smaller servings are clear: smaller portion sizes can allow you time between servings to digest your food and therefore feel fuller. This is one of the best ways to feel fuller on less, but you can also experiment with different foods to experience the sensation of feeling full without overeating.

Feeling fuller on less: You can work to decrease your portions while encouraging your body to feel fuller on less in a number of ways. The easiest method is just to put less on your plate. Even if you end up eating two or three plates of food, it is less likely for you to overeat. This is because, when we load our plates with food, we feel obligated to eat everything on our plate. If there is a small amount of food on our plate, it is easy to eat and then consider a second serving, whereas with a full plate you may not be hungry halfway through but force yourself to eat the rest. This can lead to overeating, so be sure to limit the amount you take at the beginning of a meal in case you misjudge how hungry you are. You can supplement this by using smaller plates, which physically limit how much you can actually take. Alternatively, you can put a small amount of food on a large plate and spread it out to make it look like more food than it actually is. When you finish the serving, your mind will see the large, empty plate as representative of finishing a large meal, which will decrease your subconscious need to eat more. You can use this technique with beverages as well, using taller glasses to make yourself think that you drank more than you actually did. These techniques draw on our understanding of subconscious visual cues that we discussed earlier. Another psychological technique to feel fuller is to place a mirror in your kitchen or dining room so that you can see yourself as you eat. By watching yourself consume your meal, you become more aware of the food that you are putting into your body in real time, therefore making yourself feel fuller faster. By using mental signals, we are able to feel fuller on less. Studies also suggest that chewing food longer contributes to feeling fuller—you can even extend this technique after meals and use sugar-free chewing gum to help curb cravings. Caffeine also helps decrease hunger as an appetite suppressant, but you should be wary when introducing more caffeine into your diet, as it can quickly become very unhealthy. Try having a regular cup of coffee in the morning and then a small cup after lunch to take the edge off of any hunger urges while not suppressing your natural need to eat.

You can also change your diet to include foods that are more filling. Certain foods make you feel fuller than others; for example, the number of calories from oatmeal is more filling than the same amount from ice cream. If you follow this to its logical conclusion, you will find that less oatmeal makes you full than more ice cream. The word used to describe feeling full after eating is called satiety. A satiety index measures the fulfillment you get from certain foods (on a scale) and rank them in their ability to satisfy hunger. Foods with a satiety index high than 100 are considered more filling, while foods ranked below 100 are considered less filling. This is helpful because knowing what foods rank with a higher satiety index can help you consume fewer empty calories and feel fuller after a meal. The satiety index is determined by protein content, fiber content, density, and energy per unit weight. Foods high in protein and fiber help you feel fuller for longer by affecting satiety-related hormones and increasing digestion time. The density of a particular food is used in reference to the amount of air or water contained in it, which can increase the level of satiety. The energy per unit weight tells you the number of calories for its weight—foods low in calories for their weight are more filling and are usually low in fat. Boiled potatoes rank very high on the satiety index, with a rating of 323. Compared to most other foods that are high in carbohydrates, potatoes are incredibly filling, and they are a good source of vitamins, minerals, protein, and fiber. They also contain very little fat. Other foods with high satiety index numbers include:

- Eggs — Try healthy options like poached or boiled eggs as opposed to fried or scrambled eggs.
- Oatmeal — Make plain oatmeal interesting by serving it with stewed fruit.
- Fish — As mentioned before, salmon makes for a healthy and filling meal.
- Soups — Vegetable soups and stews make great comfort food, especially in the winter or when you are sick. Plus, they are super filling!
- Lean meats — Avoid fatty meats in general to increase satiety.
- Greek yogurt — Add fruit or granola for

breakfast or a healthy snack!

• Vegetables — Vegetables can be served alongside the main course or constitute a meal by themselves. Experiment with vegetables that you may not have tried before and look for exciting new recipes to spice up your diet.

• Cottage cheese — It works great as a healthy side dish.

• Legumes — Beans are some of the most versatile foods and can be added to almost anything!

• Fruit — Like a sweet addition to any meal or as a snack by itself, fresh fruit is a healthy, natural alternative to other sweet foods.

• Quinoa — If you have yet to try quinoa, let its incredibly high satiety index ranking convince you. Quinoa can be used as an alternative to rice or mashed potatoes in a meal.

• Nuts — Various nuts make great snacks. Try making your own healthy trail mix at home by using your favorite nut varieties!

• Popcorn — Stove-cooked and lightly salted popcorn is a delicious and surprisingly healthy snack. Go easy on the butter, or leave it off completely!

On the other hand, there are many foods, such as ice cream and croissants, that have very low satiety index numbers and should be avoided when trying to feel fuller on less. In general, stick to foods that are high in protein and fiber, are less dense, and pack fewer calories per unit weight.

Now that you are equipped with the information of when to eat and what to eat, you will truly have the chance to personalize and adapt your healthy eating diet plan. As mentioned before, if you started with one diet plan but now wish to pivot to another, that is perfectly acceptable because it is an example of growth in your understanding of your body's needs! As you alter your diet, change your mealtimes, or reorganize your kitchen supply, you should celebrate all changes as evidence of the advancement of your healthy eating mindset! As always remain mindful and aware, especially when safeguarding against mindless overeating. However, if you find yourself slipping out of the present and turning to old habits of mindless snacking, do not punish yourself or feel guilty. Everyone "fails" or makes a mistake at some point in their life, and most people fail every day. The negative attitude toward failure is completely unwarranted because failure is actually a gift—mistakes allow you to learn from the past and give you the opportunity to improve and try again. It can actually be very cathartic to address your perceived failure directly and even share it with others. Remember your network of support—this is where they are needed the most. Call up a friend or meet with a family member and explain what you have done. Tell them about how you have been working so hard to improve your mindset and health, and then talk to them about how you slipped up. Explain how it feels and why it is so important to you to keep trying. Asking for support and encouragement is extremely empowering, and your supporters will no doubt feel honored that you confided in them. In turn, they will give you plenty of love and support so that you can get back on track and keep improving. Also remember that, just as there is no single path to success, there is no single definition of "failure." To put this into perspective, you should realize that what you may consider a mistake in your journey, someone else may think of as a regular break from their journey. In relation to this, remind yourself that each journey is taken at a different speed. If you find yourself falling into mindless munching every once in a while, it may seem like you are delaying your journey to a healthy eating mindset and may never get there. However, as we have discussed, there is no true "end" to a journey of growth, and so you can never really sabotage yourself or put yourself behind schedule. With this in mind, take comfort in going slow and gradually becoming acquainted with your needs. For the most part, the reality of the world is unchanging, so the time it takes you to come into full awareness, and consistent mindfulness is actually a bit irrelevant. Put all of this into perspective and allow yourself to relax into the present. All of these minor successes and setbacks are working together to cultivate your mindfulness, and so none of it can be ignored or blown out of proportion. Building off of this understanding, take a little confidence in yourself and cheer yourself on every time you find yourself refocusing on the present and adopting an aware and positive mindset.

CHAPTER 6: MEDITATING ON FOOD

The best way to improve your relationship with food is to just appreciate food for what it is. Food is delicious, it comes in many forms, and it can even be the basis of relationships or appreciation of entire cultures. Take time to simply enjoy food rather than worrying about weight or peripheral health concerns. We are not trying to use food as a tool—we want to improve the way we think about food in relation to ourselves. To begin meditating on your relationship with food, begin by appreciating the sights, smells, and tastes of your favorite foods in order to form new, positive connections with it. Go to a market and look at all the fresh fruits and vegetables and appreciate their beauty. Eat out at a restaurant and marvel at the way the chef plated the meal. Appreciate the visual beauty of food and try to connect that beauty to the act of eating—in a way, you are taking that beauty into your own body. How wonderful is it that you essentially get to eat art?

Next, consider getting your hands dirty and really appreciate the texture of food. Explore the tactile nature of food and discover the unique textures of fresh fruits and vegetables. As you prepare your food, take time to revel in each step—from peeling vegetables to slicing up meat. When you eat your food, appreciate how the texture changes from before to after cooking, and consider the difference in feeling between touching with your hands and experiencing the textures of the food in your mouth. Savor each bite and let each different taste linger. Is it salty, sweet, sour, bitter, or savory? The Japanese word for "savory" is umami, which directly translates as "deliciousness." What are the different aspects of deliciousness, and how are they present in the food that you are eating now? How does the aroma complement the taste? Does the scent of a certain food bring back memories of cooking with relatives, or does it make you think of a special meal you had at your favorite restaurant years ago?

Psychologists say that smells are closely linked to memories, and you can use these associations to develop your new healthy relationship with food while paying respect to your old connections. Relish in the different smells of a prepared meal versus its original ingredients—can you still smell the fresh herbs? What does your meal sound like? Does the light clinging of silverware in a restaurant comfort you, or do you prefer the quiet buzz of a meal in the fresh night air? Do you remember what the market sounded like when you bought your ingredients? What are your favorite sounds of food and cooking—the sizzling of meat, the soft slices and thuds as you cut up carrots, or the way that your chewing sounds louder in your own head as you eat? Delving into this deep appreciation of food helps you develop your relationship with eating, engaging your mind as you feed your body. This is what it means to "meditate" on food.

Holistic Healthy Mindsets

Creating awareness of your mind and body while cultivating an appreciation for food is the very heart of a healthy eating mindset. However, becoming aware of your health and actions while continually reminding yourself to focus on the present not only improves your relationship with food—it also impacts all aspects of your life. This is what is called a "holistic" healthy mindset. There are many ways to approach holistic health, and healthy eating is one such gateway. It is only natural for healthy improvements in one avenue of living to echo to other parts of your life. As you develop healthy habits and awareness in your healthy eating mindset, you will turn to other ways to improve your health and quality of life. This is another reason why the journey to a healthy eating mindset is never-ending—it continues to evolve to include other parts of your life. Once you improve your relationship with food, you may seek to improve other things related to your body through the mindfulness techniques that you learned here. For instance, you may take the idea of the food diary and transform it to become an exercise log. The healthy improvement afforded by exercising, of course, help improve your physical health and can be related to the food you eat. This makes it an obvious choice for inclusion in your healthy eating mindset. In addition, now that you understand how emotions can affect your appetite, you may seek to better improve your mental well-being by seeing a therapist, getting more involved in the spiritual aspects of mindfulness, or asking a friend to join you on your mindfulness journey, therefore creating a new social bond based on emotional and mental well-being. Perhaps most importantly, you can also apply the personal and private lessons that you have learned about healthy consumption on a community level, encouraging others to utilize the farmer's markets or even working with others to establish a community garden. The network of support that we identified in Chapter One may even become the basis of a new social bond among you and your friends, and you can enrich your health and theirs through social support. In this way, a healthy eating mindset draws from all parts of your life and then enhances them in turn. Therefore, the healthy eating mindset is a two-fold holistic mindset—it accounts for holistic health while also improving holistic health.

Mindful Eating Techniques in All Aspects of Life

The techniques that you have learned in order to cultivate your healthy eating mindset were presented in direct relation to eating and appreciating food. However, these techniques often draw on other activities and aspects of your life, such as exercise, social interaction, and hobbies, and are necessarily connected to those other parts of your life. Once you have begun to incorporate these other aspects into your healthy eating mindset, it is only natural to turn the flow of information and energy around in order to impact these other aspects of your life positively. That is how mindful eating techniques can be incorporated into activities that seemingly have no relation to food or eating. This constant growth of your healthy eating mindset into other areas of your life will sustain your new mindset and allow it to remain fresh in your mind. As a never-ending journey, you may find that you have to keep moving your goal. This is great news! It means that you have come further than you ever expected. Just think: by simply raising your awareness of your mind, body, and the work that's around you while supplementing that awareness by making a few small lifestyle changes—you had grown immeasurably from when you first picked up this book. This growth is rooted in understanding and commitment, and the growth can continue forever as long as you are willing to continually look for ways to improve your health and quality of life. In order to do this, you can simply go on as you have been for the entirety of your journey, staying focused on the present while keeping your goal in mind. Look for ways to incorporate mindfulness into everything you do, while always turning your experiences inward to promote growth. Experiment with using techniques learned from your healthy eating mindset to supplement growth in your personal relationships, career, and community.

Slowing down: Slowing down when eating allows you to meditate on food in a deeply thoughtful and appreciative way. It can reveal things about food that you had never realized before, creating the opportunity for discovery of yourself as well as the foods you enjoy. It also helps you feel fuller as you chew more and eat less. It raises awareness of your physical and emotional state, connecting the two and informing your perception of your relationship to food and your increasing physical and mental health. Taking time to slow down and engage in mindfulness techniques to raise awareness of your thoughts and actions is key to sustaining your new healthy eating mindset. Just as you cannot rush the journey, you should not rush any aspect of your life. Slowing down in all activities can help you better appreciate your relationship between mind and body or body and activity. The more you consider the small movement of your body or the places that your mind goes when performing regular activities, the more you are able to discover about yourself. Slowing down helps you cultivate a relationship with all things, whether it is your car as you are driving, your friends as you are talking to them, or your home as you go about cleaning it. Whatever you are doing, take a moment to slow down and simply experience what it is like to live and move in the present. Perhaps you will learn something new about an activity that you have been doing for years, like discovering that you actually enjoy washing the dishes because it helps you feel responsible while allowing you to function without having to think very hard about what you are doing. The awareness that you have cultivated in relation to food will trickle into other relationships that you have and other activities. This is part of why a healthy eating mindset is necessarily a mindset of holistic health.

Mindfully questioning: As we have developed our mindsets, we have discovered many methods of bringing awareness to our actions and encouraging mindfulness in all that we do. Going forward, you must continue to be mindful of your actions—questioning your choices and the steps that led you to where you are now. Just as you have explored the influences of your thoughts, emotions, and actions, be vigilant and understanding of the influences present in other people's lives and the world at large. Perhaps now you can mindfully question what your next step will be. Your journey has been deeply personal and unique so far but also guided by the information outlined in this book. From this point on, you will be the chief informant of your actions. In a sense, you are venturing into uncharted territory. You must be sure to mindfully consider all of your actions and choices in order to discover the best path for the rest of your journey. Will you have a traveling partner? Will you head off in a direction you previously avoided? How will your path transform? Perhaps, you walked for the majority of your journey, but now you wish to run. These metaphorical choices can be used to guide your future choices, but in the end, the decision will be yours alone. While you weigh your options and approach exciting new places in your psyche, always remain mindful, aware, and considerate of yourself and others.

Putting your health first: Throughout your journey, overall well-being has been emphasized over weight-loss or toning your body. This is because changes in your body are merely effects of changes in your overall health. Realizing this was part of the development of your healthy eating mindset. As we discussed with diets, focusing on your physical appearance often overlooks your physical health and generally neglects your mental health. In order to address weight and fitness in a healthy way, you first focused on your relationship with food in order to improve your physical and mental well-being. If you have found that you have lost weight over the course of your healthy mindset journey, then you should consider that an effect of altering your mindset rather than the accomplishment of a major goal. That being said, the healthy eating mindset should have increased your appreciation for your body and improved your body image, so you are likely to benefit from any weight loss in a healthy and mindful way rather than reducing all your growth to a physical change. Similarly, as you extend your healthy eating mindset into other areas of your life, you should always put your health first and before any improvement in body shape, social standing, or wealth.

Incorporating Other Activities into Your Healthy Mindset

A healthy eating mindset does not need to be limited to patterns of consumption. You can also incorporate other activities in order to improve your overall health and your relationship with food. Taking up a hobby can have a major positive impact on your mental well-being, and you can use this information to benefit your healthy eating mindset directly. For instance, many psychologists have endorsed the activity of art therapy as a way of improving self-expression and communication, and it also helps you create methods of creation in order to balance out destructive thoughts. Some art therapists have identified art therapy as especially helpful for those who suffer from eating disorders such as bingeing. Monsters or oppressive abstractions often represent negative feelings toward a patient's relationship with food, and collages of food in paintings can represent the conflict that arises when a binger desires food but knows that they are engaging in an unhealthy habit and cannot stop. Art therapy allows such people to deeply explore their emotions and exercise their ideas about themselves and their eating habits in a safe environment. This, in turn, allows them to put their internal thoughts into perspective and examine their feelings in a tangible way. The process helps patients to articulate what they want to say about their condition without fighting for the right words, therefore allowing them to express themselves in a cathartic way. Art therapy is used in such a way as to help the patient reevaluate their relationship with food and move forward in a productive way. Since there is already precedence for art therapy helping to improve relationships with food, you might also consider incorporating painting or drawing into your life as a way of further exploring your healthy eating mindset. Here are some art therapy exercise responses that you can use at home to further improve and sustain your healthy relationship with food through painting or drawing:

• Paint, draw, or make a collage depicting your healthy eating journey!

• What kind of food are you craving right now? What else in your life are you craving, and how can you connect the two visually?

• What is a food-related memory that you have? When we discussed scents and memories, did a specific image come to mind? Alternatively, think of a person or a moment in your life and illustrate the memory using pictures of food.

• How do you feel about eating? Create an abstract visual representation of your feelings about food.

When you have finished your art therapy project,

consider discussing it with someone close to you in order to fully explore the feelings you experienced while making it and how you feel looking at the finished project. Also, try to experiment with some other activities to improve your healthy eating mindset, and then return to art therapy to visualize how those activities have helped you.

Gardening: What better way is there to improve your relationship with food than growing a harvesting food yourself? If you did not opt to adopt the garden-to-table diet plan option and start a garden of your own, now is the second-best time to do so! You do not need a huge plot of land or any fancy machinery to start and maintain a garden. You can start a small private garden in your backyard, in pots, or in your window box—or you can get involved in a community garden. Research shows that gardening on any scale can massively help improve mental health, which makes it an excellent addition to your healthy eating mindset. Cultivating vegetables and taking care of plants helps gives you a sense of responsibility while also allowing you to practice a nurturing mindset. This kind of beneficial experience can translate to helping you improve your social relationships in addition to your relationship with food. Gardening can also help you feel more connected with the world, particularly with other living things. While feeling connected, you can relax and feel at peace in your life, encouraging mindfulness that allows you to understand your place in the world and also exist in the present. Finally, gardening can be a natural way of dealing with built-up stress, allowing you to direct that energy into a productive activity. In summary, gardening can vastly help improve your mental well-being, and it can also help you save a little money by growing some of your own vegetables and herbs!

Travel and Food Tours: One of the best parts of traveling is the opportunity to try new things, not the least of which should be new kinds of food! Travelling can be beneficial because it allows you to get away from everything for a little while. Everyone can use a vacation every so often, so why not take one in order to improve your healthy eating mindset? A fun way to incorporate travel into your new healthy eating habits is to travel to a place where you can sample authentic food that you enjoy or want to try. This can be somewhere far away or close to home. Once you have identified where you want to go and what you want to eat, look into booking a food tour so that a local expert can show you all the best eateries around. Traveling and tasting new foods can be very fun on your own, but you may benefit from taking a friend along for the ride. The best part about traveling while trying new foods is that you get to experience the culture and the people. This will help you feel more connected with the world while also providing you with an exciting and one-of-a-kind experience! There is really no way that you can go wrong with a vacation and food tour, and both activities can greatly benefit your healthy eating mindset. You may even discover a new aspect of healthy eating during your travels!

As you can see, the healthy eating mindset permeates into all aspects of your life and also draws from all of your activities and experiences. The best way to support the constant growth and improvement that comes with sustaining a healthy eating mindset is to constantly look for new activities to include in your healthy lifestyle. Whether it is something as small as taking time to deeply meditate on food once every day or as massive as taking a vacation out of the country to experience new food and new cultures, there are many things you can do to supplement your new healthy eating mindset and improve your relationship with food. Drawing on earlier discussions of experimentation and variation in relation to the growth and improvement of your health, you can see that there is no single way to explore this never-ending journey to a healthy eating mindset. As long as you are staying present, maintaining awareness, putting your health first, keeping the mind-body connection in mind, and focusing on constantly improving your relationship with food, there is no wrong answer. Congratulations on cultivating your healthy eating mindset!

CHAPTER 7: BEYOND DIET – HEALTHY MINDSETS FOR EVERYTHING

When we began this journey, we started with the understanding that healthy eating is more than just diet. At the heart of this statement is the emphasis on a healthy mindset before anything else. Now that you have successfully cultivated a healthy eating mindset, you may wonder what else a healthy eating mindset can help improve. The good news is that a healthy mindset in one area of your life can easily be applied to other areas of your life as well. There really is no bad news! Once you are comfortable with the improvement that you have seen in your eating habits and relationship with food, you can begin exploring other aspects of your lifestyle that would benefit from mindfulness. Perhaps you will choose to pursue activities that directly help in maintaining your healthy eating mindset, or you might explore other avenues of expression and improvement. Whatever activities you decide to engage in, be sure to take that same level of awareness that you learned to adapt in your healthy eating mindset journey into all the areas in your life that you choose to explore.

Mindful Cooking

Similar to gardening, mindful cooking can help improve your relationship with food while also benefitting your mind and body. Mindful cooking is simply being present and aware as you cook. Being aware of your ingredients, tools, and your hands as you put everything together and work to create a meal can help you better appreciate the art of cooking and bring positive energy to the activity. The key is to simply enjoy the act of preparing a meal and receive joy back. Try using the guided meditation technique that we discussed the last chapter—take in all the aspects of cooking with all your senses. Smell the aroma as you bring a pot to boil and feel the heat of evaporating water on your neck and face as you stand over the range. Allow the sound of the knife on the cutting board to resonate throughout your body, feeling the vibrations through your hands. Let no detail go unnoticed or unappreciated. You want to experience everything about what you are cooking rather than falling back into mindless action and distraction. The goal of awareness in cooking is to establish a stronger connection with the food that you are preparing and cultivate that relationship into something meaningful for you. This will further enrich your experience of eating the food, thereby nourishing your healthy eating mindset. Stay present and intentional in your actions, thoughtfully carrying out all the steps without letting your mind wander to other things. Focusing on your actions and creating awareness of your body and the space that you are working within helps intensify and direct your energy into your cooking, making it more enjoyable and rewarding. Mindful cooking should make you happy and bring you peace, allowing you to channel your energy into the food that you make, therefore creating meals that reflect your thoughts and emotions.

Take cooking lessons: If you want to be even more adventurous with your mindful cooking, try taking cooking lessons! This will be especially rewarding for novice cooks, as lessons will teach you the basics of cooking and allow you to appreciate the art itself better. Cooking class can even be fun learning moments for experienced home cooks! Getting out of your comfort zone and trying a cooking class will expose you to new recipes. You may have an old family recipe for a certain dish that you swear by and would never think to change. But if you learn a completely different recipe in a cooking class for the same dish and it turns out actually quite tasty, you may consider adopting a few things here and there. This will encourage experimentation and variation, which are important aspects of a healthy growth mindset. You will also meet new people through cooking classes, and you may even form strong, lasting friendships. It is much easier to make new friends through shared interests than through random encounters—so if you enjoy cooking, you are likely to get along well with other people in your cooking class! If you enroll in a cooking class with multiple sessions, eventually, you are likely to encounter a particular food that you have new tried before. Tasting a new dish is an interesting experience in itself but attempting to make that food using an unfamiliar recipe makes the entire experience an entertaining and fascinating journey for you and your classmates! This is another instance of experimentation and variation being brought into your life, which shows just how effective a cooking lesson can be in fostering new aspects of your healthy eating mindset. On the other hand, if you choose to attend a one-time cooking lesson, you can turn the entire affair into a date night with your partner or a fun outing with friends. If one or more of you are less than experienced in the kitchen, this is sure to create lasting memories of humorous moments, not to mention allowing you to share your food-related discoveries with others. Some more practical benefits of cooking lessons include teaching you new techniques to use when cooking, introducing you to seasonal or regional recipes, as well as providing you with healthier options of what you can cook. After taking one or more cooking lessons, you will be able to incorporate what you have learned into your mindful cooking so that you can continue to nourish your healthy eating mindset.

Mindful Exercise

For many people, diet and exercise go hand in hand. Although we do not wish to minimize the many wonderful benefits that exercise has on your overall health, this book did not focus on exercise because it approaches healthy eating from the position of a healthy mindset above all else. However, once you have established your healthy mindset, you should be more than ready to engage in healthy, mindful exercise. If you did not regularly exercise before embarking on your mindfulness journey, yoga is a great place to start. It is a highly accessible activity that you can do in the comfort of your own home with little to no equipment. You can also easily find beginners' yoga classes in most cities if you wish for more structure and a social element. Other popular exercises that complement a healthy eating mindset are jogging, swimming, and strength training. The reason that exercise is so important to overall health is because it reduces the risk of heart attack, helps manage your weight, moderates your blood pressure, lowers your cholesterol, decreases the risk of type 2 diabetes and certain types of cancer, strengthens your bones, joints, and muscles to prevent injury or lower the risk of osteoporosis, improves sleep, and gives you more energy. Physical activity also has important mental health benefits such as treating depression, reducing negative thoughts and feelings, releasing stress, increases opportunities for social bonding (if working out with others), improving your general mood, and increasing levels of serotonin and endorphins in the brain, which are naturally produced chemicals that make you feel happy.

Join a sport: Just like taking cooking lessons, joining a local recreational sports team, or getting involved in a sports club can be physically and mentally rewarding while teaching you new things. Intramural or community sports make exercising fun and social, and they benefit your health just as much, if not more, than going solo at the gym. When playing a sport, you have more motivation to work hard than when you are simply following an exercise regime. Competition in sports gives your workout a purpose and also requires you to keep up with your team members. The benefits of working in a team do not stop there, though. The socialization created by sports teams helps you develop relationships with others and also increases your confidence and sense of well-being. In addition, the nature of recreational sports is that they do not require the intense commitment that is associated with professional sports. This ensures that the activity is kept fun and light-hearted. On top of these benefits, playing recreational sports also provide you with all the benefits of general exercise, including improving overall physical health and positively impacting your mental well-being. If you have been thinking about joining a sports club or have long admired athletes but never been involved in sports yourself, now is the time to take the plunge, especially since you have grown while developing your healthy eating mindset and can further improve through physical activity!

Mindful Sharing with a Mindful Community

Now that you have experienced the benefits that a healthy eating mindset can bring to a person's life, you may finally go out and share that positive experience! One of the best and most productive ways to share your positive experience is through volunteering. Humans are social creatures who are naturally generous and genetically predisposed to want to help others. This is why volunteering and donating feel good. Often, the more we give to others, the better we feel. This may sound selfish in a convoluted way, but it is actually just positive biological feedback. We encourage ourselves to help others, and it is incredibly rewarding when we do. Volunteering increases our happiness and confidence because it allows us to help our community while also satisfying our innate need to give to others. All of this creates a natural sense of accomplishment in ourselves and a desire to further help our community. Volunteering can also enrich our social lives—thus connecting us with other volunteers and making friends with both the people we work with and the people we help. As we work to improve the community, we also work on improving our relationships with others and our social skills. Studies also show that volunteering positively impacts our mental well-being by actively working to reduce the effects of stress, anxiety, and anger in our everyday lives, combating depression by bringing happiness into other people's lives, and providing you with a sense of purpose, especially if you choose to volunteer regularly. With all the benefits that volunteer work brings to both you and the community, it is an excellent way to share all the positive energy that you have cultivated through our mindfulness practices!

Volunteer at a soup kitchen: There are many people in the world who cannot provide themselves or their families with the nourishment that they need. By taking time out of your busy schedule to help feed these people, you are sharing your positive experiences and healthy mindset with those that need it most. The act of helping others also enriches your spirit through the transference of positive energy and a sense of community building. Volunteering, in general, is a very rewarding experience—and volunteering in a way that directly relates to your healthy eating mindset can help reinforce all the positive changes that you have made in your lifestyle recently. Doing volunteer work at a soup kitchen or other organizations that provide free food for people in need will allow you to work according to your abilities and according to others' needs. For instance, if you enjoy cooking, preparing the meals will let you release positive energy into other people's lives while also edifying yourself. If you would rather serve the soup and chat with the visitors, you can bring joy and light into people's day while also satisfying your need for social interaction and positive feedback. Other ways that you can volunteer to help charitable organizations like these include fundraising, organizing events, and getting the word out into the community through advertisements.

Donate to your local food pantry: Similar to volunteering at a soup kitchen, donating canned goods and non-perishable items to your local food pantry also helps community members in need while providing you with all the mental and social benefits of volunteering. Donating to a food pantry is especially well-suited to the healthy eating mindset because it asks you to consider all the food resources available to you in comparison to the few resources that many other people have available. Consider mindfully taking stock of your pantry at home and choosing foods that are easily accessible to you but difficult to come by for lower-income families. Also, take the effort to raise your awareness of other items that people need and food pantries accept. Non-food items that are welcomed at food pantries include toiletries like deodorant, soap, shampoo, toilet paper, shaving cream, toothbrushes, toothpaste, and feminine hygiene products, as well as cleaning products and childcare items like diapers. Once you have evaluated all the unopened food and non-food products you have available, try taking a little bit of everything to donate to a food pantry. You can put everything into bags or boxes and set them in your car so that they are ready to be donated the next day. If you desire, you can also go out to the store and buy new products to donate if you do not wish to deplete your supply at home and can afford the gesture. When you get the chance, bring all of your donations to the food pantry of your choice. Further mindful actions to take include helping the food pantry volunteers unload your donations, sort them, and then store them in the correct places. If you would like, you can also use this time to ask about volunteering at the food pantry. If you would like to get more involved with what the food pantry does but cannot manage to make time for volunteering, consider starting a food drive to collect donations for the food pantry. This is easy to do, and you can simply place a large box next to your desk at work or another place with a sign that clearly states the purpose of the food drive and where the donations will be going. Spread the word to friends, family, and colleagues so that everyone can get involved in your food drive. Once you decide to end your food drive, take all the donations to the food pantry and help them sort out the different items. They are sure to be very thankful for all your hard work!

In addition to volunteering and donating in order to support and enrich your wider community, be sure to return to those who supported you throughout your mindfulness journey. Part of being mindful of your place in the world and in your immediate community is acknowledging the flow of energy from one person into other, from someone into you, and from you into someone else. Be mindful of these dynamics and seek to do your part to nurture the positive energy in yourself and others. The best way to do this is to identify the people who have helped you along your way to growth and to return the favor.

Thanking your network of support: Now that you have successfully developed your healthy eating mindset, it is time to return to your network of support that we establish in Chapter One in order to thank them for being there for you. In a sense, this is the action that truly brings us full circle in our mindfulness practice. If you found support online, be sure to post an update about the success of your healthy eating mindset journey and share some tips and words of encouragement for those thinking about following your example or engaging in a healthy lifestyle transition of their own. Similarly, be sure to inform your friends and family about your journey in person. Consider taking your support network out for dinner in order to celebrate your success and thank them for their encouragement. Find other ways to give back to your community of friends and family, sharing your mindfulness and positive energy to show them how much you have changed and how much you appreciate their support. Of course, if any of your friends or family members choose to pursue a healthy eating mindset journey of their own, make yourself available as a resource for them, and volunteer yourself as a ready and willing member of their own network of support.

As we near the end of this book, remember that this does not mean that your journey must also come to an end. You are encouraged to continue seeking growth and improvement in all areas of your life—not the least of which is your healthy eating mindset. Share your experiences with others and encourage them to make healthy changes in their lives. Set an example by always working to improve yourself in mind and body.

CONCLUSION

Thank you for making it through to the end of Healthy Eating Mindset! Let's hope it was informative and able to provide you with all of the tools you need to achieve your goals—whatever they may be.

The next step is to implement the mindfulness techniques introduced in this book into your life, taking the first step toward reshaping your relationship with food. This book should have provided you with all the information you need to plan and prepare for your healthy eating journey successfully, and it is sure to help guide you if you find that you have any questions along the way. Once you begin your journey, you should be able to understand the connection between the mind and the body in such a way that makes it simple to develop your new healthy mindset with a food diary and healthy diet plan. If you encounter emotional trouble on your journey, you will be able to overcome any setbacks—thanks to your new understanding of emotional eating. In addition, the awareness that you have cultivated about your actions will help you curb any mindless overeating that you may have experienced in the past. As you learn to feel fuller on less, you will be able to take your time and meditate on your relationship with food—finally cementing your healthy eating mindset as the perfect confluence of mind, body, and sustenance. Once you have developed your healthy eating mindset, you can bring further awareness to all aspects of your life and work toward cultivating a healthy mindset for everything!

Hopefully, this book has successfully introduced you to the positive benefits of a healthy mindset, as well as how it can drastically improve your relationship with food while increasing your physical and mental well-being. Once you have accomplished this change in your eating mindset, you should be equipped to address all kinds of healthy mindset changes!

Finally, if you found this book useful in any way, a review on Amazon is always appreciated! Thank you very much, and best wishes on your journey to a healthy eating mindset!